What's Possible?

Ayurvedic Odyssey:
The year yoga changed my life.

Mary Roberts and Karta Purkh Singh Khalsa

LOTUS
PRESS

Box 325, Twin Lakes, WI 53181 USA
email: lotuspress@lotuspress.com
website: www.LotusPress.com

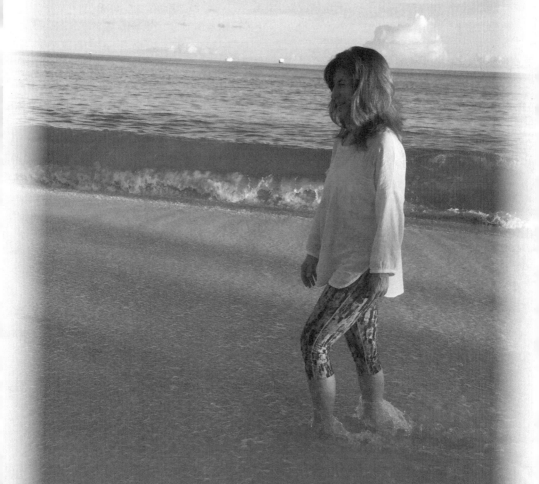

62 Years Young
Mary Roberts' Story of
Ayurveda, Yoga and Transformation
May 1, 2015 - May 1, 2016

First Lotus Press Edition 2018

ISBN: 978-0-9406-7648-0
Library of Congress Control Number: 2018940520

Printed in the United States of America

Cover photo taken by Srinivasan Orel Revivo

For information address:

LOTUS
PRESS

Lotus Press
Box 325, Twin Lakes, WI 53181 USA
email: lotuspress@lotuspress.com
website: www.LotusPress.com

This book is dedicated to my mother,
Virginia Marie Dragich,
who was my first teacher in this life.

CONTENTS

Foreword ix

Introduction xi

What is an Ayurvedic-Yogic Lifestyle? 1

Nothing Happens By Chance 5

When NOT to trust your inner compass? 13

Love-Hate Relationship with Food 21

Basics of the Yearlong Study 31

Settling in at the Ashram 39

Battling with Myself 51

Hurricanes and Storms Within 63

Six Months Milestone 73

Six Month Milestone - Commentary *79*

Lighting Us Up 83

Saint Makers 99

Enuresis - Commentary *115*

Nearing the Finish Line 137

Results 153

Results - Commentary *156, 161*

Before & After Photos *163*

Resources 171

Gratitude 175

FOREWORD

by *Karta Purkh Singh Khalsa*

Living Ayurveda and using Ayurvedic herbalism can keep you well. With this knowledge, you can achieve balanced health, a priceless gift. Imagine a time in the near future when you're free from sickness, when you haven't been bothered by even a painful joint or uncomfortable bloating for a long, long time. That future can become your reality.

I've seen thousands of patients regain vibrant health, and for my entire adult life I've been involved in the revolution that is transforming the health care system in America. Ayurveda and yoga play a big part in that. I am sure you, like other Americans, want to know what you can do to protect yourself from the degeneration, aging and daily irritations that undermine the quality of our lives.

If you have relied on conventional treatments and they are failing you, learn yoga and incorporate Ayurveda in your life, starting today. In this book, you will read about the success story of an admittedly typical American woman who did just that. Committing to the historically potent herbal traditions of India, fused with a modern slant, she found transformation. This could be you. I hope you take to heart what she says about her experience. Admittedly, she spent the year in a concentrated yoga and Ayurveda environment, but there is so much you could do in your own kitchen.

As an Ayurvedic doctor, herbalist, nutritionist, yoga teacher and educator, I have been making Ayurvedic approaches palatable to the modern mind for almost fifty years. I have seen people like you reap extraordinary benefits and reprieve from a vast range of health concerns by making these principles part of their lives. For the first thirty-two years of my career, I was the apprentice of an Ayurvedic master, Yogi Bhajan. Not a day goes by that I do not thank him and this outstanding legacy for allowing me to witness the transformations I have seen and been privileged to be a part of. Most important, I have raised 3 children in Ayurvedic style, and lived to tell about it.

Ayurveda is the ultimate self-care system, especially when it is fused with yoga. Natural healing is all about prevention, and the techniques of Ayurvedic self-care are geared toward bringing you back into balance quickly and effectively, so that you don't have continued symptoms. Ayurveda has a different vision of the healthy human. Think not just the gradually failing, getting through the day human, but a vibrant being with energy to excel. You'll see that in detail in this book when you read Mary's (Padmavati's) story.

You've noticed that there are myriad natural healing theories and methods. And that they all seem to conflict with each other. How could they all be right? They can and they are. But no one regime works for everyone. Individualization is the key. We are born into different bodies, each with a different heritage, and we have all lived different lives. Ayurveda has worked out the idea that people are different and need to be treated differently. And it has worked out techniques to do just that. It is a coherent, cohesive theory that gives us a measuring tool that people can master and apply. It explains the reason some people get better on one diet and others tolerate different foods. The overarching concept of energy balance is the glue that holds all the techniques together. In this book, you will see that Ayurveda is systematic, organized, and straightforward to learn. We will put it in perspective. The wealth of information in this book makes sense. We hope it inspires you to action.

INTRODUCTION

What's a woman like me doing in an ashram?

In 2015, I began the unlikely adventure of living an Ayurvedic-Yogic lifestyle for one year at the Sivananda Ashram Yoga Retreat in the Bahamas. The aim was to discover "what is possible?" physically, mentally, and spiritually when a typical Western lifestyle is traded for a traditional Eastern lifestyle.

I was honored and fortunate to be guided by Karta Purkh Singh Khalsa, an Ayurvedic Doctor who is one of the foremost natural healing experts in North America and has been practicing Ayurvedic medicine for more than 40 years.

I was also blessed to do this study at the beautiful Sivananda Ashram Yoga Retreat in the Bahamas. The spiritually and energetically supportive environment provided an ideal, controlled setting to discover, "What is Possible?".

Banyan Botanicals, a provider of certified organic Ayurvedic herbs, agreed to provide the herbs and supplements prescribed by KP Khalsa with which to start my journey. They continued to support the study for the second half of the year by substantially discounting the cost of my herbs and supplements.

I am grateful for the support of KP Khalsa, Sivananda Ashram Yoga Retreat and Banyan Botanicals. Each graciously agreed to support me in this yearlong project without requiring or requesting any commercial endorsement.

To readers who are skeptical that a lifestyle change can result in improved health, be assured that the clinical results and my personal experiences are presented as accurately as possible. I immersed myself in daily living at the Ashram devoting many hours to the study and practice of Sivananda yoga and Ayurvedic principles. I completed yoga teacher training and additional course work to enhance my understanding of Ayurveda.

It is my hope that from my stories and the results of the study, that you may find inspiration and hope for your own life.

I truly believe that having the physical ease of movement and strength to live your joy and your purpose is not just for someone else, it is for everyone.

It all began in 2014 at an Ayurveda workshop led by James Tennant at the Tejas Yoga Studio in the South Loop neighborhood of Chicago. I had never heard of 'Ayurveda' before, yet was very intrigued. Later, when I had the opportunity to visit an Ashram in the Bahamas as a vacationer while at the same time attending the annual Ayurveda conference held there, I didn't hesitate. But more on this later.

At the time, I had no idea what an Ashram was. The Sivananda Ashram website described it as, "*a spiritual learning center, where students and practitioners go to study, practice, and live in a devotional community.*" To me, it sounded much like a monastery found in Western cultures. However, the website photos of yoga classes held on the amazing beach, and lush greenery and flowers were nothing like my idea of a monastery. Upon arrival I was delighted to find the ashram to be as beautiful as the photos. I learned that it was not made up of just a couple of temples on the grounds of a secular yoga retreat. The ashram was the entire five-and-a-half acres.

Quite unexpectedly, this one week vacation turned into a year-long study that is the basis of this book. Not in my wildest imagination would I have dreamed up the adventure I am about to share with you.

Why was this adventure unlikely?

I am a mainstream Midwestern woman with Eastern European roots. My children are happily married and starting their own families. I cherish my roles as Mom and Grammy and welcome any time I get to spend with my children and grandchildren.

I was living in a beautiful condominium building in the upscale Prairie Historical District in downtown Chicago. I had wonderful family and great friends in the area. I was plugged into an amazing local yoga community and great organizations like Landmark, Rotary One Cosmopolitan, the United Nations Association, and Seagull Institute. I enjoyed yoga, walks on the lakefront, dinner and drinks with friends, professional meetings, dancing and partying until all hours. Having my own business gave me the flexibility of working from home and setting my own schedule. Whether in my role as mother, employee or entrepreneur, I set high standards for myself and give 100%. The 'work hard and play hard' image of an ambitious urban professional woman aptly describes how I lived my life. I had freedom, independence and a fluid schedule. It was a lifestyle I enjoyed immensely.

As was typical of suburban families in the 1950's and 1960's, I was raised on an abundance of meat and highly processed convenience foods. Since my teen years, I was a yo-yo dieter. I adored ice cream, candy, pizza, chili cheese fries, hot dogs, nachos, and plenty of meat and seafood, along with red wine, margaritas, and chocolate martinis. But soon I'd feel lousy and the pounds would creep on. I've tried most fad diets, only to slip back into eating all those high calorie foods again. Even as I eventually eliminated the ice cream, chili cheese fries and dairy products in order to be 'healthier' and control weight, my daily eating habits included skipping meals regularly and eating all the day's calories in one meal which was usually dinner.

I also experienced sleeping problems. On a typical day, I would stay up late, often past midnight, and then struggle to fall asleep. The quality of my sleep was poor and fitful, and I would wake up in the morning just as tired as when I went to bed. My coffee, the stronger the better, served as my wake-me-up energy drink of choice. As many people I knew had similar sleeping and coffee habits, these issues seemed quite normal. Coffee in particular, seemed to me to be a necessity of life.

Unlike Liz in Elizabeth Gilbert's book and subsequent movie "Eat, Pray, Love" I was not going through any existential crisis. I had not become a puddle on the floor, sobbing incessantly and crying out "What Should I Do, God?". There was no voice from within telling me to withdraw from life. Yet, I was continually seeking answers about a higher purpose and the meaning of life. I wanted to know what more I was destined to do in this lifetime.

Yoga and Ayurveda sparked an intense interest that I needed to follow. It was like that intuitive pull I get when I meander into a bookstore or library. Thousands of books and dozens of topics can be unappealing to me and not merit a look, while one or two sections draw me in. I investigate each a bit until one or two books pull me in so intensely that there isn't really any decision to be made. I need to read those books. This journey was like that. Yoga and Ayurveda would not be ignored. I had to learn more and see where they took me.

Then I arrived at the Ashram where no caffeine, meat, seafood, eggs, or alcohol are allowed. The lacto-vegetarian diet that is served is designed to promote good health, harmony, balance, and calm. It is a very different approach to food and eating than the "eat for fuel and for fun" style that I was accustomed to. Also, I'd be living in a tent hut and using communal bathroom facilities, making my multiple routine bathroom trips quite the challenge.

When I wrote my BestYOU blog entry about 'the leap' shortly before the adventure all began, it read:

"This leap I was about to take, felt similar to when I was a young girl, all smiles inside and heart completely open to whatever this new journey would bring my way.

Any of my fears and nervousness had to do with being able to juggle all the balls of a move out of the country - lots of loose ends to deal with and many logistics with my housing situation and my belongings and selling furniture and address changes etc.

The actual leaping to Sivananda Ashram Yoga Retreat and the year of living an Ayurvedic - Yogic lifestyle - while not at all a logical decision, I was truly excited about the discoveries that lay ahead."

Being part of a study really intrigued me, and I was open to this new challenge. Throughout the book, you will find my journal entries to be in italics with the dates noted. I journaled daily during the year at the ashram. The entries are not polished and edited, as this book is about sharing my journey with you. Please excuse the occasional misuse of words and less than perfect grammar. Raw and real, I've learned, are important. They point us in an inward direction.

As I write and share my very personal stories with you, know that my heart is wide open and full. I feel honored and privileged that you are spending your precious time in reading this book. I deeply hope that you will find it to be of benefit to you. Thank you for joining me on this journey.

Namaste,

Mary

WHAT IS AN AYURVEDIC-YOGIC LIFESTYLE?

When diet is wrong, medicine is of no use.
When diet is right, medicine is of no need.

Ayurvedic Proverb

Yoga is the journey of the self, through the self, to the self.

The Bhagavad Gita

I've studied Ayurveda by listening to and reading the experts over the past couple of years. I am a relative newcomer to the study of this vast science, but here's what I've learned:

"Ayurveda means the 'Science of Life' ("Ayur"= life, "Veda"= science or knowledge). It is the traditional medicine of India and the oldest system of health care in the world. Ayurveda is concerned with both preventative and curative medicine. According to the College of Ayurveda in California website, "it is at least a 5,000 year old system of Natural Healing, and perhaps as old as 10,000 years. During India's time of foreign occupation, Ayurveda was suppressed."

More recently, both in native India and throughout the world, Ayurveda has been enjoying a major resurgence. Tibetan medicine and Traditional Chinese Medicine have their roots in Ayurveda, while early Greek medicine embraced many concepts originally described in the classical Ayurvedic medical texts that date back thousands of years.

And despite its beginnings in these ancient times, Ayurveda is one of the *most advanced herbal sciences in the world.* It is a system that provides guidelines on ideal daily and seasonal routines, diet, behavior and the proper use of our senses in order to achieve perfect balance, and therefore health, in body and mind. Everything from types of food, colors, aromas, sounds, meditation and even touch are used to create this state of harmony.

In Ayurveda, there are five elements noted as being in all living things. Ether, air, fire, water and earth are the building blocks of life. These elements unify us, and the three doshas, or fundamental energies that are composed of the five elements, determine our physical and mental characteristics that make each of us unique, depending on the proportion of the dosha expressions.

Each person has a basic body type, like a blueprint of our physical and mental characteristics that can be broadly classified based on three doshas, called Vata (air), Pitta (fire) and Kapha (earth) in Sanskrit. (For those new to Yoga, Sanskrit is one of the oldest, if not the oldest language known. In India and Southeast Asia, Sanskrit is much like Latin and Greek in the Western World. It is a language still used for religious ceremonies, and it is the language of Yoga).

A quick introduction of Vata, Pitta and Kapha follows, as I'll explain the doshas in more detail later on in the book.

Vata types have more of the air and ether elements, with their qualities of dryness, coolness, roughness, and mobility. They tend to be on the thinner side, are more delicate, and can never seem to get warm. They are creative and can be a bit spacey at times, while being picky eaters and quite sociable.

Pitta types, made up of more fire and water, are consequently heated and intense - hot, sharp, quick, and light. They have a large appetite - they literally burn food quicker than other types - and can easily tend toward extreme behaviors.

Kapha types have more of the earth and water elements, with qualities of heaviness, dampness, coolness, and smoothness. They are nurturing and work at a steady pace. They enjoy more sedentary activities and are content with low levels of activity - as a consequence, they sometimes also have difficulty maintaining their weight.

Something I personally like about Ayurveda is the focus on the individual, noting that each person is unique with a distinct path for optimal health. It is not a 'one-size fits all' solution to physical and mental health issues, nor is it a 'take a pill - quick-fix' lifestyle. The Western approach of 'one pill' for all headaches or 'take this drug' for depression determines the treatment based on the specific ailment, not based on the specific individual. Drug makers create meds that are for the mass population, whereas in Ayurveda, any treatments that are prescribed focus on bringing balance to an individual person.

When the body and mind are in harmony, normal physiology is maintained or restored and healing, if needed, is able to take place naturally. Nature creates the meds, as all naturally grown food has medicinal qualities. The goal of Ayurveda is a balance and integration between the environment, body, mind and spirit.

It's worth noting that all the Ayurveda experts at the conferences I attended at the Ashram in January 2015 and 2016 were adamant that, if you get into an accident or break your arm, Western medicine and surgical procedures are absolutely the way to go. However, once you've been stitched up, an Ayurvedic approach to restoring balance and harmony in the body, mind and spirit will be the most powerful aid to healing.

Healing with Ayurveda also incorporates Yoga, and living a Yogic lifestyle includes adhering to the principles of Ayurveda. The two sciences are part of a singular system that leads to health, well being and balance.

Yoga is defined as the union of the mind, body, and spirit with the Divine. Swami Vishnudevananda, a direct disciple of Swami Sivananda (the master yogi and saint that the Sivananda Ashram Yoga Retreat was named for), developed a simple approach to classical yoga, specifically for those of us he was called to teach in the West. Sivananda Yoga is a synthesis of the ancient wisdom of Yoga in five basic principles, which can easily be incorporated into everyone's own pattern of life. He states in his book, titled *The Complete Illustrated Book of Yoga*, that, "It (Yoga) shows the way to perfect Health, perfect mind control, and perfect peace with one's Self, the world, nature, and God."

The Five Points of Yoga taught by Swami Vishnudevananda are as follows:

1. Proper Exercise (Asanas) – Asanas are Yoga poses that help develop a strong, healthy body and mind by enhancing flexibility, especially of the spine and improving circulation.

2. Proper Breathing (Pranayama) – Deep, conscious breathing connects the body to its battery, the Solar Plexus, where tremendous potential energy is stored, thus reducing stress and many diseases.

3. Proper Relaxation – Relaxing helps cool down and recharge the body, keeping it from going into overload mode and easing worry and fatigue.

4. Proper Diet – Eating simple, pure, natural vegetarian foods that are easy to digest and assimilate and have a positive effect on the mind and body, as well as limiting the impact on the environment and other living beings.

5. Positive Thinking and Meditation – These conscious controls of the mind are the true keys to achieving peace of mind and eliminating negativity in our lives.

My year of living at the Ashram would focus on adhering to the principles of both the sciences of Ayurveda and Yoga. I was a true novice and would be learning these principles as I went along. I had no idea what was in store for me. I just knew that it felt like a good and healthy path, and I was willing to be open to whatever showed up and to experience it as best I could.

What is Possible? was the basic question I focused on throughout the yearlong study. That question often helped me persevere when I wanted to give up. I couldn't pick and choose whatever I felt like doing, or give any less than my best effort, if I really wanted to find out "What is Possible?". I had chosen the lifestyle to explore, the environment to conduct the study and the experts to guide me.

Staying true to the study of an Ayurvedic-Yogic lifestyle, and whatever that meant, was my goal.

NOTHING HAPPENS
BY CHANCE

Evolve. Expand. Grow.
Man is not a creature of circumstances.
His thoughts are the architects of his circumstances.

Swami Sivananda

On December 14, 2014, an email from a dear friend started a chain reaction that led to an experience that seemed inconceivable for me at that time.

The summary of the message - *I know you are interested in a yoga retreat. Have you heard of this place? I've been there. www.sivanandabahamas.org.*

After checking out the website and noting that there was an intensive one-month teacher certification training program, I was definitely interested in finding out more. I'd been considering yoga teacher training for nearly a year, and on that very morning, I had filled out the application for the program from my local yoga studio. Previously, I had hesitated to sign up for the local training because of the yearlong commitment of Saturdays required to complete the course. I finally decided to go for it and planned to turn in my paperwork the next day. Surprisingly, the cost of the immersion program in the Bahamas, including food and accommodations, was the same as the cost of the teacher training program at my local studio back home.

Pure Chance?

As I browsed through the Sivananda Ashram website, I was almost giddy with excitement and filled with a sense of possibility. As well as the yoga teacher training immersion, they offered an Ayurveda Conference in January, and the opportunity for yoga vacation programs. It was a dream come true for me - and all in the Bahamas!

I recalled that I hadn't yet used the generous birthday gift given to me by my brother's family - a roundtrip airline ticket on SouthWest Airlines. Even though I doubted the possibility, I anxiously checked the website to see if SW flew to Nassau. They did, having recently added the route for seasonal flights. Lucky me!

More Chance?

I wrote a few emails back and forth with my friend who mentioned the yoga retreat in the first place. She spoke of the specialness of the place, and knowing that the airfare was taken care of, things were falling into place. Within a few hours, I had registered for the Ayurveda Conference in mid-January, reserved my room for a week, and booked my flight to the Sivananda Ashram Yoga Retreat in the Bahamas. I had never heard of Sivananda yoga, had no idea what an ashram was, and had never been on a yoga retreat. I was going alone, and the only available space was a shared bedroom with a community bathroom. I did no usual Google search to compare other places and prices, nor the usual querying of friends and family. This was quite unlike me. I was not someone who leaped without doing due diligence. Yet, somehow I was compelled to make this spontaneous decision, and even more surprising was how good I felt about it. I held off turning in my application for the teacher training at my local yoga studio. I had until the end of January to register, and the excitement of this new possibility was taking my full attention.

When I arrived at the ashram on Paradise Island, I was filled with anticipation and wonder at the ease with which this trip had materialized. After a delicious dinner and meeting a few other vacationers, I made my way to my room. I barely finished unpacking in time to go to the satsang (morning and evening gatherings for meditation, chanting and lectures) - but I did make it, and to tell you the truth, I had no idea what was happening on that first night.

Arriving at the large, open-on-the-sides platform where satsang was held, I saw that most people sat cross-legged on cushions on the floor, while others sat in chairs along the side. There were large pictures of what I learned eventually were deities and the founders of the Ashram, as well as other yogis. The pictures were hung on brightly colored, material-draped walls at the front. There was also an altar with small statues and flowers. The look of it seemed very strange to me.

I learned that 'satsang' was the Sanskrit word meaning 'in the company of truth'. Satsangs brought together all those at the ashram for meditation, chanting, spiritual teachings and lectures. That first night, after meditation, 300 or more people chanted *Jaya Ganesha* (the opening chant or prayer done at every satsang) with *Hare Krishna* chanting infused throughout, accompanied by the harmonium, tambourines, small drums, clapping, and small cymbals.

I closed my eyes and thought, "Hare Krishna????" "WHAT am I doing in a place like this?"

I kept picturing the Hare Krishnas at the airport, in their long robes, with shaved heads and braided strips down the center of their heads, handing out leaflets with smiles on their faces.

> *"I feel like a fish out of water, with darkness hiding much of the property until morning. And the satsang chants were unfamiliar and foreign sounding to me ....I consciously noted my judging of the shrine and large dedication photos to founding yogis, and then chanting of Hari Krishna, with people clapping and playing various instruments all around the room - was really uncomfortable." (Jan 15 journal entry).*

With eyes closed during the entire chant - and it is a long chant - I kept repeating over and over, 'stay open, don't judge', 'stay open, don't judge', 'stay open, don't judge', 'it's only a week', stay open, don't judge'.

> *"Still uneasy about the strangeness of satsang the evening before and worried about not hearing the wakeup bell, I slept lightly but comfortably, the first night. I had the room to myself, which was a nice bonus - though a roommate could arrive any day...*
>
> *The bell is quite loud and near to my area of rooms - so I heard it no problem.*
>
> *5:30 am is really early, but I am determined to experience the full yoga retreat offerings.*
>
> *25 minutes of silent meditation after the prior night of sitting yogi style, or trying to, for 2 hours, was tough at 6 am in the dark of the early morning. But, I survived and kept lifting my chest in inhalations to sit straight.*
>
> *Then chanting that same chant as last night and a few others and then an interesting lecture - all BEFORE 8 am.*
>
> *It rained on and off throughout the day, so yoga could not be done on the beach platform. It was lovely to hear, see, smell the rain while we did our poses.*
>
> *I attended 2 yoga classes, two workshops that had yoga and lecture combined in each, went on an 11 am tour of the ashram and barely fit in a shower - was busy all day." (Jan 16).*

By the second night, in satsang, I kept my eyes open and found myself swaying a little to the chanting of *Jaya Ganesha.*

By the third morning, I had read all of the translations and realized that the chant basically praised God in many names, from Krishna to Jesus to Buddha to Mohammed and more. I didn't know much about the deity names like Ganesha, Saraswati, Siva or Rama, but from what I read, I understood that the chant was joyful and all about devotion to God.

> *"A little easier to get up this morning - sitting is still tough and feeling stiff this morning. 8 am yoga on inner water platform was fun and lovely - sun shone through palm tree'd blue skies. The yoga instructor was amazing and all my kinks were gone as the class ended...I met some nice, new people...*
>
> *I was starting to learn the opening chant and could mimic back some of the phrases quite easily. By the evening satsang, I was starting to listen to and find the opening chant less foreign. I noticed more of the enjoyment of others chanting, rather than critiquing the experience.*
>
> *Looking forward to start of the conference tomorrow evening and booked an Ayurveda massage treatment Shirodhara with hot oil - should be relaxing and a new experience." (Jan 17).*

The first three nights I was there, the evening satsangs provided beautiful music as part of the Spiritual Music Festival, and included an incredible Iranian singer, a lively Christian Gospel singer, and a Rabbi who led Jewish chants. "Unity in diversity" is a major belief at the ashram, and I found the different types of music quite interesting and enjoyable. The quality of the programs was excellent.

One of the women I met on the first night was leaving the Ashram midweek, and she asked if I had a business card so that we could keep in touch. When I handed her my card, she immediately noted that the beaches on my card looked like the Bahamas. Not having paid much thought to my business cards background photo until then, I looked closer, and sure enough, it certainly appeared to be our Paradise Island beachfront - amazing!

Another incidence of Chance?

The Ayurveda conference and week at the ashram went by quickly. I felt refreshed, invigorated and relaxed all at the same time.

> *"The beautiful weather made for a lovely day - water was multi-shades of blue - just beautiful. I feel peaceful and engaged and relaxed as I am getting better acclimated to schedules and locations of things and yoga routines - food is very much to my liking, but I'm hoping to relax my appetite a bit - not accustomed to the ravenous feeling since I began the vegetarian diet changes - and so much yoga and pranayama*

breathing contribute to the hunger I think, plus the 2 meals a day - all a bit different to adjust to." (Jan 18).

"Walk on the beach meditation was amazing - peaceful and beautiful - my favorite satsang of the week.

Relaxing hot oil treatment and massage with Kaddha was wonderful and felt so nice.

Met more new people and a roommate arrived today - Susan from Michigan." (Jan 19).

"Susan is lovely and fun to have a roommate." (Jan 20).

I'm not sure why or how it happened, but by the end of the week I was happily chanting along during satsangs and loving every minute of it. It felt so nice to have the constant presence and naturally flowing songs of God as a daily part of this life. There was nothing conscious about what was happening and how I felt. Somehow the yoga shook something up, deep inside me. And it felt good.

"The time has come for me to leave this beautiful place. My spirit, body and mind have been nourished and strengthened. The ocean feeds my senses in an amazingly peaceful and yet powerful way.

The Ayurveda Conference speakers inspired me and further ignited my interest in the art and science of life that is Ayurveda. The yoga teachers have been skilled and patient. My practice has grown and balance is strengthened. I've learned so much with nearly 4 hours of yoga practice a day, and I've loved it! Today, in the headstand workshop, with Ambika, I learned the headstand with no need for a wall.

As I sit writing this, I am breathing in the last moments of loveliness and a young woman is playing a ukulele and singing on the beach front. The ocean breeze is blowing my hair, and the beauty of the colors of water and nature are all around me.

One last walk on the beach and then the journey homeward. I know I will be back here - I Love it and how I feel :) Om." (Jan 22).

While flying back to Chicago, I decided to do my teacher training at Sivananda Ashram Yoga Retreat. I didn't know when, but I knew I'd be back there. The first morning after the trip, full of enthusiasm, I began researching my return right away. There was a teacher training that would begin on February 4. I called the ashram to see if there were any private tent huts left and if I could register for the course, but there was only one tent hut left and they would not hold a course space for me until I had my flight booked. When I then checked the flights, they did not prove easy to book - no flights on SouthWest, with holiday season past and prices on other airlines had increased substantially.

Things were not flowing easily, like the last time. So, for once, I decided to let it go, do nothing, meditated a bit on the ashram and just waited.

The idea of doing a yearlong Ayurveda study in the controlled environment of the ashram came after several days of this new approach of meditating, clearing my mind, not pushing, and just letting it be. One morning I awoke with my brain flooded with possibility. I found that I was consumed with sharing more about Ayurveda with everyone. The wonders of the science seemed so amazing and simple to me, that I felt like I needed to investigate as deeply as I could and share whatever helped me with others. The concept in my head was clear and fully developed, as though I'd been working on it for weeks - and of course, I hadn't.

My idea was to take an initial complete physical inventory, including eye exams, using Western scientific methods, plus do an Ayurvedic assessment. I'd then track progress, take monthly photos, journal daily, blog about the experience each week and collaborate on the writing of a book, showing the results at the end. I also was inspired to take yoga teacher training and training in Ayurveda as part of the year-long plan. I realized that I was a beginner yogi and would be relatable to the mass population. I thought, "I'd want to read a story about someone doing this project for a year."

For the study, I would follow all the directives of the Ayurvedic expert in an effort to see "What is Possible?" for a mainstream American woman with a host of typical health issues like sleep deprivation, addiction to strong coffee, digestive problems, constipation, loss of hand strength, hearing loss, hair loss, scalp cysts, cracked and dry feet, knee problems, neck stiffness, joint issues and more.

I wrote an email note to Karta Purkh Singh Khalsa (KP), who was one of the presenters at the Ayurveda Conference in the Bahamas. There had been hundreds of people in his evening talks and 50 or more in his workshops. He didn't know who I was, and certainly wouldn't know my email address. I knew it was a long shot. As an internationally recognized speaker and expert, best case scenario in my mind was that I might hear from him in a couple of weeks .

Yet I heard back from KP's office the very next morning.

More Chance?

The note said KP was intrigued. An initial meeting was set up with his assistant Sat Pavan, and then I completed the writing of my proposal and sent it directly to KP. A meeting was scheduled with him via phone, and within weeks, KP had agreed to collaborate on the project.

"My insides are dancing and my heart feels warm! There is an actual tingly sensation that I feel in my skin. I am crazy excited over the new adventure that is now full speed ahead in the planning mode. Yay!!

The meeting today with KP Khalsa confirmed our collaboration and his full support of my proposal to live a year Ayurvedically at the Sivananda Ashram Yoga Retreat with him as my guide throughout the journey.

...What an extraordinary day!" (February 12)

Next, I reached out to the Ashram. There is a Karma Yoga Immersion Program that involves contributing service to the Ashram for 6-7 hours per day for a minimum of 3 months, with tent accommodations, food, yoga and attendance at satsangs provided at no charge. There was no mention of the possibility of a year long stay on the website. However, when I spoke to Rukmini, a senior staff member of the Ashram, she said they needed someone to work in the marketing department, preferably on a more permanent basis than the standard three-month stay. Once she was sure that I really wanted to experience the Karma Yoga (selfless service) and seriously devote myself to a year of life in an Ashram, she welcomed me. The timing was uncanny, as I would be needed on May 1st for training before she, who would be my supervisor, left for 6 months to go to Israel.

It just so happens that my background was in marketing and communications -

More Chance?

I had just enough time to provide the required 60-day notice of my departure to my landlord. When I signed my lease the prior July, not knowing why and without any plans to move, I had asked my landlord if it would be ok with him to include the possibility of an early termination of my lease. It was agreed that, if I gave 60 days notice, the lease could be terminated up to three months early. April 30th was the soonest I could end my lease without penalty. How perfect was that?!

Another Chance happening?

I spent the next two months preparing for the trip, giving away and selling all my furniture and condensing my belongings to about a dozen boxes and some hanging clothes that my mom graciously allowed me to store at her home in the suburbs of Chicago.

Next, I reached out to Banyan Botanicals to see if they would be willing to provide me with herbs and supplements in support of the project. It wasn't an immediate answer, as they had a process to go through in considering such a request, but after a couple of weeks, they said Yes! They provided the first six months of product to launch me, and then gave me 50% discounts on the remaining purchases I made. They even signed up and followed my blog throughout the year.

The flow of everything seemed so natural and easy.

Or mere Chance?

My son, daughter-in-law and my little 10 month-old grand-baby moved to another state two weeks before I left for the Ashram and took some of my bigger furniture pieces for their new home. I was delighted about the furniture, and their moving seemed much less difficult for me with my own adventure in the planning stages.

Chance?

My daughter and her family, who live in London, were able to visit a week before I left for the Bahamas, as my daughter had a business trip come up in Chicago. And her baby - my other grand daughter - would have her 1st birthday in September which, as it turned out, was perfect timing for me to travel to London. 90 day Visa permits are the limit in the Bahamas. Re-entry to the country after a few days' departure was the routine for those of us staying longer than three months, and my grand-daughter's birthday would coincide perfectly with my Visa trip.

More Chance?

Everything was aligning for a smooth journey. I felt it at the time, but I now know with every fiber of my being that God led me on this year-long journey. There is no voice to this knowing. I can describe it best by saying that when I got on the path I was supposed to be on, it felt like a river flowing with ease. Many of my prior paths felt like uphill climbs and struggles all the way. I learned from those uphill climbs, but I could have learned the same lessons while flowing down the river.

I had so much more to learn.

WHEN <u>NOT</u> TO TRUST YOUR INNER COMPASS?

The Purpose of human life is to be Happy.
Pain is natural; suffering is optional.

Buddha

My strong streak of perfectionism, natural competitive tendencies, and my need to succeed were amplified in the work environment in which I spent a large portion of my adult life. Any uphill struggles were met as challenges, and the unrelenting pace of it all just enticed me to run faster. I didn't realize it then, but the path I was on was not a good one for me, mentally or physically.

In most of our workplaces, we are well aware of the preference for thought leaders that leave their emotions out of decisions and preferably far from the office. As a consequence, I spent years downplaying emotions and feelings, while up-selling my intellectual skills. My first career after receiving my university degree was as a teacher. While I think it is important for teachers to display some feeling, they also need to keep most of their personal emotions in check to maintain control in their classroom. One of my professors even recommended that we should not smile until Christmas. He suggested that if the students were afraid of us, they would listen better as we taught them. I didn't take that advice, and I very much enjoyed teaching, only leaving that vocation to raise children.

As an at-home Mom for my next life choice, emotions were displayed freely. This was a wonderful time of life, and I treasured the luxury of staying at home with our children.

Raising and teaching children came naturally to me and was fun! It was definitely exhausting and challenging too, but the overriding memories of that time are of laughter and happiness, and while God and Christian teachings were mainly reserved for Sundays, the basic principles of kindness, honesty, compassion and fairness were a part of our everyday life.

However, as is the case in 50% of marriages in the U.S., I was destined for divorce. I've spent hundreds of hours analyzing and contemplating the 'what happened?' and 'how did it happen?' and 'why did it happen?' and 'who was at fault?' questions. Now, I can sum it up in one word - karma - and it's nice to finally be detached from the burden of the constant wondering. For me, there is little else left to say about that particular topic, although I will say quite a bit more later about karma.

Following divorce, it was necessary for me to re-enter the workforce. Although I had been an at-home Mom for nearly twenty years, I was civically engaged, and had served in numerous positions on a number of community boards. I had also been elected twice to the school board in one of the largest districts in the state, where I served as Vice President and President. Neither I, nor my mind, had been idle. Yet the volunteer world is very different from the professional workplace.

After the trauma of my divorce, I buried deep personal emotions, read voraciously to fuel my mind, and rolled up my sleeves in preparation for a world of work. And I can admit now, I was unsure and nervous about whether I could succeed. At the time, I wore my armor of confidence and went full steam ahead. I definitely followed the 'fake it, until you make it' philosophy. Yet deep down inside I was scared to death of failure.

It was also a time of upheaval in the Catholic church as revelations of child abuse by priests filled the headlines. Being a child advocate and the mother of a son, I was appalled by this, and my reactions to these revelations were those of anger and disgust. I was already in an unhealthy emotional and mental state, coping with divorce. Church rules about annulment proceedings initiated by my former husband infuriated me further. As a result I was unforgiving and extreme in my response. While our children had benefitted from a wonderful Catholic college preparatory high school education, I stopped going to church, except on holidays, and began to feel very negative about the Catholic religion in general.

When a friend I knew through work committed suicide because he no longer was able to cope with the past he endured as a victim of abuse by a priest, that was the final straw for me. I was extremely angry with the Catholic Church and its leadership that, in my mind, had allowed abuse of our young, impressionable children.

At the time I returned to work, my daughter was away at university, and my son was pretty self-sufficient. For the first couple of years, however, I worked part-time, so that I could still attend all the sporting events, band, chorus and other activities that my son was involved in. I had attended all of my daughter's important school activities and I was determined to do the same for my son, even as a single mom. I began working full time when my son left for college and luckily, the modular construction company I worked for was growing rapidly and welcomed my full time employment. I enjoyed working, but long, stressful days, lack of sleep, and excess food and drink were the norm for me at that time. I thought I was balancing those negatives with regular running and periodic weight lifting. I maintained a moderate weight and appearance of fitness for many years.

I had no idea how unhealthy I really was and ignored any warning signs, even when I got them. Hangovers? Everyone I knew had them. Trouble sleeping? Just the norm. Indigestion and constipation? Pretty common. Injuries that refused to heal, hearing loss, and hand strength loss, I explained to myself as simply getting older. It was as though I was on a never-ending treadmill, and as long as I wasn't falling off the treadmill it felt normal and fine. I could pretty much push myself to keep up the rapid pace. I believed I was in control. I wasn't even sure anymore if God was watching.

My inner compass was a complete mess. My imbalanced lifestyle produced signals that were no longer about health, but rather about maintaining the status quo that my mind, body, and spirit had become accustomed to. I was grateful for having a job, generally had a positive attitude, and had a history of a strong work ethic in my family. I grew up believing that hard work yielded success, and if there was work that needed to be done, I could and would do it. And rather than me or anyone else questioning it as being unhealthy or possibly too much for me personally, my action-oriented, can-do spirit was generally admired, especially by employers. In the U.S. especially, long days, few breaks, eating lunch while working at our desks, and few vacations are the norm.

However, about 10 years ago I was diagnosed with pinched nerves in the base of my spine that quite severely incapacitated me, and even mere walking was accompanied by shooting pains down my leg. My sciatic nerve was screaming out with every movement. I wanted to avoid the surgery that I was told would likely be necessary after I tried pain medication, physical therapy, massage therapy, and went to a chiropractor and pain specialist. I even had an MRI. Nothing that was prescribed by the numerous doctors I saw worked for more than a few hours at a time. The pain specialist suggested cortisone shots directly into my spine, and if that didn't work, then surgery was the only remaining solution.

I was emotionally and mentally a wreck, trying to lead a normal life by continuing to work while in constant pain. Outwardly, few people even knew I was struggling with health problems. I wore my mask of 'everything's just fine', while I tried to cope on my own. Eventually, as a last resort, the excruciating pain and immobility led me to yoga.

Yoga, after a few months, dramatically relieved the pain, and within 6 months, it eased the pain completely, without any surgery.

You might guess that yoga then led me to good health - but not really - at least not without plenty of setbacks. I did what most of us do. As soon as the pain started to subside, I increased my pace of work and social life again. I still did yoga regularly, but instead of 3-4 times per week, I dropped back to 1-2 times per week, most weeks, and occasionally skipped a week or two. On average, I maintained a once-a-week yoga routine. Not exactly a route to health and fitness.

Of the 168 hours in a week, I spent 1 hour and 30 minutes doing yoga for my health.

Now, having practiced yoga every day for over a year, I think that statistic is pitiful, but back then, like most people, I thought it was normal and even laudable. Running was no longer part of my regular routine because of my injury, and to compensate, I changed my eating to less caloric foods and skipped breakfast and lunch most days. My inner compass was so messed up that this sounded like a reasonable solution.

I enjoyed working at the small company that a team of us grew into a thriving business. I learned a great deal, wore many hats, and we all worked extremely hard. I thrived on the constant and ever-changing demands of the work, and felt needed. I was running so fast on the treadmill of life that I found it hard to see that there was any way other than my way. Naturally, when I was offered a government position that was quite a step up from my role with the startup company, I accepted.

Rising to leadership roles meant controlling my emotions even more than I already did and displaying yet more outward determination and seriousness about my work. Government leaders are still predominantly males, and the climate is mostly male-oriented. Determined to succeed, I worked harder and longer hours than anyone on my team. When I wasn't working, I read and took classes to increase my knowledge base. I played hard too, but mostly on weekends, late at night. I was determined to reach a leadership role, a measure of success to my way of thinking. As I look back, I think I was also seduced by the power that accompanies leadership positions. I had tasted that power in my role as President of the School Board, as special privileges and treatment came with the title.

I eventually became the Director of the Office of International Trade and Investment for the State of Illinois. I was responsible for ten overseas offices, an office in Chicago and an office in Springfield, Illinois. In my role, I worked with Consuls Generals, Ambassadors and Trade Commissioners from around the world. I welcomed business and government delegations from countries across the globe, and spoke on behalf of the Governor of the State at many international events. These events were held at the finest hotels and best venues in Chicago - all quite exciting!

It was a job that I loved and felt somehow destined to be in. I worked harder than ever and was determined to be successful. It didn't matter that I had little prior international experience. Less than one month into my Assistant Director role, I was elevated to temporary Director when my boss, the former Director, resigned due to his financial dealings with a now imprisoned governor. While a sad commentary on that Governor and the Director, I planned to prove worthy of this new position.

My life became mainly work, and when I had time, occasional social gatherings with friends and family. I moved to the city and commuted daily on crowded trains. There was an energy and non-stop pulse in the city that fueled my already high-octane lifestyle. In some ways, I did well on that fast paced treadmill. I had learned the pace and just kept moving. I thought it was all very exciting and fun, and also believed that my hard work was needed, purposeful and meaningful. As Director, I worked extremely hard and put in more hours than anyone in my department. Pushing myself and others to high standards with total disregard to health was my normal, daily way of living.

The many work events and social gatherings I attended had me regularly drinking 2-3 glasses of wine every night, and more on weekends. Again, it felt normal. I rarely ate during the day, and I didn't usually have dinner until 9:30 or 10:00 pm after I got home from working. Most nights I got to bed around midnight.

I functioned fine and was not noticeably impaired or impacted by the drinking and eating patterns. I would fall asleep after tossing and turning for some time as I was exhausted, and the wine seemed to help a little with falling asleep. I would wake numerous times throughout the night, experiencing hot and cold periods and having to go to the bathroom. In the morning, I would be just as tired as I had been when I went to sleep. A couple of cups of strong, black coffee were needed to help, both as my usual laxative and to put me back into high gear for another day. And my generally optimistic attitude and push-forward nature had me greeting each day with determination and positivity.

I noticed that my skin and body were showing signs of stress, but nothing that was not usually attributed, in our American culture, to normal signs of aging. My nails were discolored, dry and had white spots. One of my injured toe nails just would not grow, and another was misshapen. Though my nails were hard, as they'd always been, they were rather gross in appearance. Weekly manicures and bi-weekly pedicures hid the 'aging'. I had an occasional Botox treatment initially, and then used fillers to build up and support my puffy eyelids and the drooping skin around my eyes and mouth. The treatments certainly had some accompanying pain, but the "refreshed and less droopy" look helped keep my spirits up. I figured it was worth it. I felt more confident when I looked rested and healthy, especially in the work environment. My professional appearance was complete with chic clothes, regularly styled hair, makeup always done, good leather shoes and purses, and beautiful scarves to complement my look. I was leading the "independent city girl, successful business woman" lifestyle that was glamorized and highly sought-after in our culture. I felt very much in control of my life.

Due to circumstances unrelated to me or my work, I became one of the victims of a political battle in the Governor's office. Out of the blue, one day I was called up to the top floor, the Governor's level of offices. I was clueless about the purpose of the meeting. I was unceremoniously given a new position, and while my pay remained the same, my role was in a different department, doing work I was over-qualified for and that I did not want to do. I had a Director title, but it was meaningless to me.

I persevered in this new role, but was miserable. Slowly, it dawned on me that I was definitely not in control. My anger and resentment were quite intensely aimed at the government leaders who I felt had forced this on me, and yet I thought I had no choice but to stay. I had a lifestyle to support, and rent and bills that needed to be paid. Plus I was unjustly treated, so I'd show them! What I planned to show them, I'm not really sure. I remained in the new position for nearly two years. It was a true inner struggle to not have a hardened heart and to not want to bury my head in the sand and just throw in the towel. I felt I had worked so hard, and yet somehow got run over by a truck and dumped by the side of the road. In an attempt to keep going, I buried those feelings and started going to yoga classes more often. The yoga helped to calm me and pass the time, as I now worked fewer hours. While I didn't realize it at the time, the yoga was also helping me to cope both mentally and physically with the feelings of inadequacy and loss that I was deeply feeling inside. The anger, resentment, disappointment, sadness and self-doubts were all churning inside, while I kept a positive face for the outside world as best I could.

I had been a mentor to many college interns throughout my career, and a number of my friends thought I was good at helping them with their problems. So finally I decided to try something new. While I was still working in government, I created a new plan and completed professional training to be a life and career coach. Feeling disillusioned with the political system and experiencing misery each day as I readied for work, I resigned from the government. I had worked five years as a teacher in Illinois, and seven years as a government employee.

I now realize that God was in control, and that once I chose to get off the treadmill, he provided me with what I needed to get back on the right path. Whether I had stayed in the job I loved or the one I hated, both government jobs were unhealthy choices for me. Who knows what health issues I might have faced if I had stayed working day in and day out in either of these situations? The good news was that I had vacation pay and unused sick days when I resigned, that ultimately helped me fund my trip to the Sivananda Ashram Yoga Retreat.

After my resignation, things started looking up. I started my own business, BestYOU LLC, on January 1, 2014 and had my first business consulting client within a month. I was contracted to be the US Coordinator for FX World Istanbul from January

2014 until the conference, which I attended in Istanbul, in October 2014. My prior role in International Trade was instrumental in my attaining that first contract with the Turkish Business Association. And on a personal level, my daughter gave birth to my grand-baby, a little girl, in September 2014. A trip to London on the way back from Istanbul to Chicago was perfect to put on my travel itinerary. It was such a happy time, and I felt such joy with my new little grand-baby's birth! It is very special to see our own sons and daughters as Moms and Dads - pure love and joy!

I also invested in myself. Having a newly flexible schedule with an at-home business, I devoted time to continuing education, and attended Landmark Forum trainings and graduated from their complete Curriculum for Living in 2014. As noted on their website, Landmark is a globally-recognized personal and professional growth, training and development company. "They are an educational enterprise that is committed to the fundamental principle that people have the possibility of success, fulfillment and greatness." I was very grateful for the powerful impact and learning that I experienced through the Landmark courses.

After my week long trip to the Ashram in January 2015, and while planning for the year-long study to start in May, other good karma (or good luck, as I saw it at the time) was unfolding. I had a new three-month coaching client, and also worked for the Seagull Institute, teaching Marketing to international students from France. Both were roles that I enjoyed immensely, and the timing of the work was ideal for my May departure.

Each step of my life's journey gave me experiences that were valuable, even though they are so different than my journey today. I hope sharing glimpses of my past reveals some of what I've been through and how I've coped. I lived as I knew how, striving for perfection, based on what I had been taught and what I had learned through the lens and values of my family and my American culture. Who I am now is a reflection of my openness to change and acceptance of that which I did not know. I've been recalibrating my inner compass through an Ayurvedic-Yogic lifestyle and the results have been, and continue to be, transformative and wonderful! It's difficult not to judge where I've been or what I've done, but my focus in noting this information is for disclosure, and hopefully as a way to better understand how I got to where I am physically, mentally and spiritually today.

When I started my apprenticeship with Rukmini, my supervisor at the Ashram, I told her that above all, I wanted to cultivate my heart. I had, for too long, buried my soft side and been the tough-minded, strong-willed, action-oriented leader who put business goals first. Health and happiness for myself and others who worked for me were a distant second. After much reflection and living for many years from my mind, I wanted something different. Intuitively, I sensed there must be a better way. I wanted to learn from and be a different kind of leader - a leader who leads from the heart.

LOVE-HATE RELATIONSHIP WITH FOOD

*Every human being is the author of
his own health or disease.*

Swami Sivananda

*Health is wealth. Peace of mind is happiness.
Yoga shows the way.*

Swami Vishnudevananda

Due to trying every diet advertised at one time or another, and having some success with them, I was never considered excessively overweight. I had an upbeat outlook on life and smiled quite a bit. Most, including me, thought that I was a model of health - as defined in America. Yo-yo weight gains and losses were my norm, and the norm for most of my friends, especially the women, who were always trying to lose 10 or 15 pounds. It was easy to tell if I had a reunion, wedding or beach trip coming up, as my weight would start going down. The actual event itself was considered a 'free day' when I could eat and drink whatever I wanted, thus resetting my body's 'normal' of poor eating and drinking habits. And the weight would gradually be put back on. Sometimes I even worked out a plan to lose more weight than I really wanted to lose, so that I could enjoy putting it back on again. As I mentioned before, my inner compass was completely messed up.

I indulged in all sorts of crazy eating splurges, usually on weekends and while watching television. I would make my way through numerous snacks, starting with what

I thought was healthy and taking it from there. Carrots and green or red peppers were a favorite start. Then I'd often decide that a little dip for the veggies might be nice, and something crunchier like crackers or pretzels would be good with the dip too. Then I might follow with a handful or two of grapes or berries. I really liked sweet and salty together. The fruit often led me to some Cool Whip or ice cream, and maybe warmed fruit on top. The ice cream would make me cold, so warm popcorn and whatever candy I had around, usually red licorice or sour patch kids or red hot tamales, might be next. When I was being 'healthier', I'd have smaller amounts of each thing I tried. Sometimes though, I ate huge quantities, and if I had bothered to add it all up, even the smaller portions were substantial. I'm not proud to share that I've eaten entire half gallons of ice cream in an evening during one of these gorges! Needless to say, I slept terribly, didn't feel very well the next day and had eater's remorse. Yet this was not a one time only occurrence. It wasn't a regular occurrence either, but still it was repeated. I knew I would feel miserable afterwards and would vow to never do it again. I kept trying different things, as nothing seemed to satisfy me. It never dawned on me that food wasn't the answer.

Not a Pretty Picture

As I mentioned earlier, after leaving my government job, Landmark education was on my path. It was at the Landmark Forum that I was able to shed my outer coating of perfection armor, and begin to look at myself and my habits more clearly and honestly.

My eating gorges were done secretly, and I had never admitted to them. What people saw me eat, and what I really ate, were quite different. Like many people, I preferred to show the outer world what I wanted them to see, rather than all of me. We grow up with visions of perfect sons and daughters, perfect students, perfect friends, perfect employees, perfect lovers, perfect spouses, perfect parents, perfect grandparents and on and on. These images are built up in our heads from the time we are little children.

Until the Landmark Forum weekend, the need to be seen in an ideal light was very strong in me. My identity was wrapped up in these images I created. Youthful, smart, energetic, happy, pretty, healthy, fun, fit - these words and more were my desired identifiers. Little did I realize that these facades were symbolic of not only an imbalanced body, but also an unhealthy and imbalanced mind.

I knew I liked the 'perfect' me better, so I figured everyone else would like 'perfect' Mary better too.

While healthy food was part of my stated interest throughout life, my reality was filled with unhealthy food choices. Everyone I knew had weight issues, sleep problems and anxiety from stress. Many also suffered from high blood pressure, diabetes, depression and other debilitating conditions. Some talked about it, others nodded in agreement, and others like me avoided the conversations altogether. Whether talked about or not, most of us ignored and just put up with the issues. For those who did seek medical help, the variety of medication that was prescribed often ended up just creating side effects to complain about on top of the original problem. TV commercials give us drug "solutions" for constipation, diarrhea, headaches, arthritis and other aches and pains. When not "curing" us, the commercials lure us to eat pizza, french fries and hamburgers, candy, beer and other sugary alcoholic and non alcoholic drinks, which more than likely would result in more drugs being needed for the effects of the junk food.

I think my favorite diet was to eat really 'healthy foods', and not much of them, during the week, and then splurge and eat whatever I wanted on the weekends. It was probably my favorite diet because it was the worst one for me. My unhealthy mind and body liked the way they were and wanted to remain unhealthy. So, the starve and gorge approach seemed perfect. If I craved chocolate cake, all I needed to do was wait until the weekend, and then I could eat half the cake or more at a time. It was party time!

Eventually I got tired of all the diets and the ups and downs of my weight, so I found another solution. I gave up dairy. Not completely at first, but I only ate it during the day. I started eating my pizza in the evening with no cheese, and I refrained from ice cream and other dairy-based desserts at night. I still snacked while watching television, but began to consider it a big slip-up when I broke my resolve and succumbed to the call of ice cream. These "slip-ups" that began with ice cream could lead to a trip to the store to buy a couple of chocolate candy bars, like Charleston Chew or Baby Ruth, and a pizza and maybe even some cookies or bakery as well - I rationalized if I was going to mess up, it might as well be a full night of dairy splurge, and maybe if I felt miserable enough afterwards I wouldn't do it again. Eventually, I did work my way into a full no-dairy diet and, unsurprisingly, I felt better. When my body wasn't being asked to digest an entire half gallon of ice cream, pizza and chili cheese fries and candy bars, all in the same day, it felt better. And that's only part of what I ate on some weekends.

My 'no-dairy' requests eventually became fashionable, and restaurants had 'no-dairy' options. I somehow felt the need to create a dairy allergy, wanting to be reassured that no butter or milk would be used in my meal, without being willing to admit that being dairy-free was my choice. It was only after the Landmark Forum that I was able to admit I did not have a dairy allergy, and instead acknowledged that 'no dairy' was merely my preference. On some level, though, I had convinced myself that the allergy was real. Admitting that it was not seems like such a simple thing to do, and yet facing one's self can be difficult.

I find this an interesting quote from American novelist, Zora Neale Hurston. "There is nothing more powerful in the outer world than to cancel your inner critic and inner judge."

The Ayurvedic View

As you might imagine, nutrition and food topics have been of interest to me my entire life.

Sadly, most, if not all of my food, digestive, sleep and skin issues were brought on by my own actions and lifestyle choices, especially the back and forth excess and deprivation cycles. Admitting that I was often eating like a human garbage can is not easy to do, but it is true. And due to my fiery Pitta constitution, my appetite has always been strong. I've been able to eat almost anything that I've wanted to eat.

Before learning about Ayurveda, and before experiencing a year-long study of a different lifestyle at the ashram, I thought any food that I chose to eat was easily and properly digested. I was wrong.

The definition of constipation - one major indicator of poor digestion - by most doctors in the the West is fewer than 3 bowel movements a week. Not once had an American doctor questioned my regularity in the past. I thought missing a day or two of bowel movements was perfectly normal. Doctors never indicated to me otherwise. And yet referencing an article written by KP Khalsa on Bowel Health, "Being mammals, we are designed so that each meal elicits a bowel movement. **Ayurveda and other natural medicine practitioners say that at least one waste elimination a day is needed for good health.**"

While coffee helped as my morning laxative, I often went a couple of days without a bowel movement. It had been my lifelong experience. My bowel movements would not have been classified as healthy in Ayurveda, as they were difficult as well as erratic and inconsistent. Besides being generally constipated, I passed a lot of gas and did a fair amount of belching - also signs of poor digestion.

Quoting Khalsa, "For people who eat healthy, unprocessed, whole food, the average transit time through our system is 30 hours. Yet, 18-24 hours transit time, according to Asian medicine, is optimal. And 48 hours is pretty common place in our Westernized society. Wondering what is the problem with the longer transit time? The end products of digestion stay in the colon, and the longer they remain, the more chance of decomposition into unhealthy compounds resulting in the development of gallstones that over time may be implicated in colon cancer."

My sleep issues, as well as my hot and cold body temperature fluctuations at night, were also signs of poor digestion. Each of these signals from my body, telling me of imbalances and less than optimal health, were shrugged off and regarded as what I'd have to put up with as I got older. And while it is bad enough that I and tens of millions of older adults are suffering, these same issues have been documented by doctors in America to be chronic complaints of young adults in their late twenties and beyond.

The experts that spoke at the Ayurveda conferences, and other nutrition specialists who presented throughout the year at the Ashram, each mentioned digestive issues as the root cause of disease, while proper functioning of the digestive system is key in disease prevention. Left untreated, those symptoms of mine that are common to so many, could lead to serious diseases such as irritable bowel syndrome, ulcerative colitis, diabetes, cancer and heart disease, to name just a few. The common phrase of 'you are what you eat' comes to mind. Our food is said to be the building block of our body at the cellular level, and the digestion of our food is important in order that the cell growth is comprised of good nutrients. Even the best food, if it is not digested properly, can form toxins in the body and manifest over time into disease. According to Khalsa, "If food doesn't get properly digested, or food waste can't get out, your perfect diet hardly matters."

In Ayurveda, all natural food is considered a good choice for someone, under certain circumstances. Foods are not labeled healthy or unhealthy as they are in America.

Instead, foods are to be chosen, limited or avoided, depending on the person's individual constitution ("Prakruti" in Sanskrit) and imbalances ("Vikruti"). According to yogic and Ayurvedic teachings, processed and refined foods are to be avoided by everyone.

During my time at the Ashram, I became even more acutely aware of my attachments to food.

Sometimes, we think that we have realized something, but the message hasn't really sunk in. It takes hearing it over and over again, in many different ways and sometimes from different people, for us to really understand it. We also need to experience it ourselves. Yoga teaches that experiential knowledge is the highest kind. Across all Eastern philosophies, there is agreement that the root of human suffering is attachment. I was certainly attached to food. That had clearly been demonstrated over and over throughout my life.

Yogis also teach that attachment leads to desires. "A desire arises in the mind. It is satisfied, immediately another comes." Yep, I had plenty of desires in the food realm.

Swami Sivananda also states, "There is no end of craving. Hence contentment alone is the best way to happiness. Therefore, acquire contentment," and "If you do not find peace within, you will not find it anywhere else."

The very first consistent improvement I noticed during the study had to do with the temperature fluctuations I had been experiencing throughout my adult life. It didn't take long on the new regimen for me to notice that my temperature was much more stable throughout the night. It was a particular blessing, since I was staying in a tent hut for May and June. While most nights were not unbearable, it was much warmer and more humid than I was accustomed to. So, the benefit of not having those periods of self-imposed body heat on top was quite significant.

With no alcohol, no spicy foods, and no iced drinks, my digestion wasn't heating up as much as it had been. When I ate a reasonable amount of food, my digestive fires also didn't have to heat up as much to digest my food intake. It all made such perfect sense, when I stopped to think about it. I was surprised, time and again, as I noticed that most teachings of Ayurveda and yoga were simple and sensible. I had the incorrect notion that ideas from the Eastern cultures were extreme, outdated and unscientific.

I was also a bit perplexed that I hadn't heard any of this information before. Why America and the West would toss aside the thousands of years of knowledge from the East, that influenced Greek medicine and Western medicine during our earlier generations' lifetime, was at first puzzling to me.

Doing a little research on the history of medicine, it became clear to me that political, religious and social pressures - not science - were the driving force of movement away from herbal medicine and the natural healing methods that had been successfully used for thousands of years. Hippocratic principles and wisdom, which Greece had probably adopted from Persia and India where medical and surgical science had always been very advanced, were in effect for 2,300 years. Hippocrates was the champion of good hygiene, but this all changed during a 1500 year long period of rejecting his ideas. Plagues and disease became commonplace. A leading physician advocating against hygiene, Galen, had been the Gladiators physician in Greece and then was personal physician to five Roman Emperors. The Catholic church adopted Galen's stance on hygiene as an old-fashioned, pagan superstition. Focusing away from the body was aligned with the church leaders' thinking at the time. Nude statues were destroyed by the church, and body washing, as well as looking at one's own nudity, were considered evidence of sinfulness and depravity. The few people who were sometimes ordered by a physician to take a bath were lowered into the tub, fully clothed.

I had wondered if the increase in life-span, that we learned was attributable to advances in modern science and medicine, could be the reason the West rejected so many of the successful treatments from the centuries-old Eastern practices. A little more research pointed to studies showing that the great increase in human life-span in the developed world (during the 19th and 20th centuries) was due to political social reforms like better sanitation systems and a return to improved hygiene and nutrition. The studies showed that increase in human life span was not due to pharmaceutical drugs or other medical interventions. There certainly were other medical advances improving infant mortality rates and contributing to better treatments to curb the spread of infectious diseases. Yet, interestingly it turns out that the American Medical Association was formed in 1847, partly in response to renewed interest in herbal medicine and the popularity of alternative medicine schools. The newly formed organization eventually became underwritten by pharmaceutical companies who had a great deal to gain. Before long, the whole medical and pharmaceutical industry turned its back on the plant world and looked to synthetic chemicals as the best choice.

By the 20th century, overwhelmed by the growth of the AMA, herbal medicine went into severe decline. Chemists learned to synthesize active plant components, and modern laboratories began to produce standardized and readily available drugs. After the discovery of antibiotics, surgical techniques were improved and modern medicine accomplished great technical advances. By the 1950's, people were accustomed to taking a pill for everything. Instead of looking at diet, lifestyle, and environment, most doctors and their patients addressed individual symptoms instead of causes. Doctors were schooled in pharmaceutical remedies and the plethora of drug solutions for illness and conditions.

Luckily, today this is changing. People are finally starting to combine modern medicine with alternative and holistic methods of healing. There is renewed interest in herbal medicine and natural healing in today's society due to disenchantment with the lack of health in our economically prosperous Western cultures. Yoga is also on the rise in the West. According to Yoga Journal, more than 36 million Americans practice yoga today, and more than 300 million practice yoga worldwide. Some say the number is more than double that. Granted, it is rarely yoga in the classical holistic sense of lifestyle, and rather more typically, it is the part of yoga that is physical exercise. Yet it is still yoga, a beginning step that will help millions of people to heal and lead better lives.

Swami Vishnudevananda, founder of the Sivananda Ashram in the Bahamas and originator of the Sivananda Teacher Training Course, was known to say that, "yoga aims to remove the root cause of all diseases", not to simply treat its symptoms as medical science generally attempts to do.

I can confirm, from personal experience, the incredible benefits of herbal medicine, natural healing and yoga, on my body, mind and spirit, after my year of Ayurvedic-Yogic living at the Sivananda Ashram.

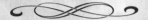

You are the architect of your own fate.
You are the master of your own destiny.
You can do and undo things.
You sow an action and reap a tendency.
You sow a tendency and reap a habit.
You sow a habit and reap your character.
You sow your character and reap your destiny.
Therefore, destiny is your own creation.
You can undo it if you like -
destiny is a bundle of habits.

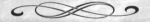

Swami Sivananda

BASICS OF THE
YEARLONG STUDY

My mission in life is to as much as possible raise the vibratory level of the world by positive suggestions and a positive way of life.

Swami Vishnudevananda

Even though living at the Ashram meant I would have no coffee, no meat, seafood or eggs, and no alcohol, I truly wanted to find out for myself: What is Possible?

I eventually learned that my health had an impact on more than just my physical well-being, but also on my relationships, those around me, and the world as a whole.

Since I was at the Ashram for the long-term, and not in crisis mode, KP and I were able to work methodically and consistently to get to the root causes of my many imbalances. However, there was a lot of trial and error, and many adjustments needed as we moved slowly forward.

Relevant Family Medical History:

> My paternal grandfather died at 73 of a heart attack.

> My paternal grandmother died at nearly 86 following several strokes and an aneurysm. She died in her sleep.

> My father had a brain aneurysm, resulting in a stroke and long rehabilitation, and died of colon cancer at 66.

My father's sister died in her early 70's of a heart attack.

My eldest brother died of kidney cancer after a 6 year battle with the disease. He was almost 53.

I have another living brother, and my mom is 86 years old.

I was a chronic bed wetter, with occasional accidents still occurring in my teens.

My list of issues when this study began:

- Vitamin D deficiency - identified in the baseline physical exam

- Erratic sleeping - throughout adulthood, usually I awoke during the night multiple times and had periods of hot and cold temperature fluctuations each night

- Constipation and difficult bowel movements

- Cracked, sore and dry skin, especially on my feet

- Loss of elasticity in skin, especially on my face but also my body

- Scalp cysts

- Thinning hair and eyelashes

- Receding hairline

- Right knee pain and sensitivity

- Left big toe nail was not growing and had been damaged for more than 10 years

- Toes starting to grow crooked and bunions forming

- Neck pain and stiffness from prior whiplash car accident

- Stiffness in shoulder area

- Finger nails discolored, yellowing and white spots and ridges

- Bloating

- Gasses passed often and with foul odor

- Belching after meals

- Loss of hearing in my left ear that was steadily getting worse

- Declining strength in my hands - I could not open jars for a few years

- Declining memory

- Difficulty finding a comfortable sitting position and also sleeping position - I was very fidgety and rarely at peace

- Frequent urination throughout the day and at night

Ayurvedic Constitution:

In Ayurveda, each of us has our baseline constitution, or body type, from the time of birth (Prakruti) and also our current constitution (Vikruti), which is affected by our current circumstances and lifestyle and often includes imbalances.

There are fundamental energies that are known in Sanskrit as Vata (wind), Pitta (fire) and Kapha (earth). Each of us has varying proportions of all three of the energies in our makeup. Understanding these three primary forces of nature (doshas) is at the core of Ayurveda. There are tests to determine one's constitution, and an Ayurvedic practitioner can provide the most accurate assessment.

KP wanted to do his own assessment when we began the study, and I had previously done a consultation with the Ayurveda practitioner at Tejas Yoga studio in Chicago. Both of these involved similar questionnaires and interviews, along with pulse readings and tongue analysis. My Ayurvedic results were consistent. My constitution is Pitta predominant with Vata and Kapha secondary, meaning my dominant energy is fire and then wind and earth are lesser energies in my makeup. When I started the study, however, I had imbalances in all three doshas.

According to Ayurveda, we have other impulses at play naturally in our lives too. The three gunas, or mental tendencies, are sometimes called 'the mental doshas'. Sattva, Rajas and Tamas are the Sanskrit words for these three gunas. Just as we all have Vata, Pitta and Kapha as part of our constitution in differing degrees, Sattva, Rajas and Tamas are present daily in our mental makeup. Sattva is purity and peacefulness, and also the impulse to evolve. Sattvic people like to progress, but in a way that is creative, life-supporting and healthy. Rajas is highly active, agitated and energetic, and also spurs questions and motivates us in life. Rajas people like to act, and their minds work constantly, tending toward impatience, impulsiveness, restlessness and high energy. Tamas is immobility, lethargic and regressive, and also sets the stage for sleep. Tamasic people like to stay the same and their mental state is more sedentary. They tend to follow set routines, are generally resistant to new ideas, and are often inactive.

I was mostly Rajasic when I began the year at the Ashram. My goal was to experience more Sattva - naturally happy, healthy and peaceful states of being.

Prescriptives:

When I started with KP, we eased into the quantities and number of herbs and supplements I would take.

The herbs will be explained in greater detail later in the book. Initially, I took the following:

- Triphala - Bowel regulation, anti-aging, overall detox and tonic

- Vitamin D3 (due to deficiency when I had my physical exam)

- Castor Oil taken with the Triphala (about a teaspoon and then increased to a tablespoon) - oil also used for daily abhyanga (body massage)

- Trikatu - Increase digestive fire

- Gokshura - Promotes healthy flow of urine

- Chyavanprash - Rejuvenation

I was also to drink a tea made of coriander, cumin, and fennel seeds, either during or right after meals. CCF tea is known to detoxify through increasing circulation and cleansing the urinary tract.

Prescriptive Recipe for CCF tea:

Tea: Coriander/cumin/fennel – 5 Tbs **dry seed mix**, brewed, immediately after each meal (can drink room temperature or cool)

Tea dose is based on daily amount, of dried herb, not volume of brewed liquid. Measure out daily dose amount of actual, dried herb. Use at least 16 volume ounces of water per one weight ounce of crude, chopped bulk herb. More water may be used, but that will make the tea more dilute, and require more total liquid to be consumed. Place herb in pan. Add cold water. Simmer, covered, for 1 hour. Strain completely (squeeze) and drink.

We ate two meals a day at the Ashram rather than three, simply because of logistics and the difficulties of having enough help to prepare meals, serve them, and clear up afterwards. I thought I would find this difficult. I was worried that I would be hungry, and I also understood that Ayurveda generally suggests three meals a day - a small breakfast, and then the largest meal at around noon or a little later, with a light meal for dinner in the evening.

However, it turned out that two meals were quite satisfactory, and I was seldom hungry mid-day.

In the spiritual environment of the Ashram, I was becoming much more conscious of my body and mind and what they were trying to tell me. I became acutely aware of the difference between actually feeling hungry and just following a schedule of eating. Having not eaten since 6 pm the night before, by 10 am in the morning, when we ate our first meal, my body and mind sent me a clear signal.

I was hungry!

I also became very aware of how the taste of what I ate impacted my appetite and cravings. Ayurveda recognizes six tastes, each of which has a vital role to play in our physiology, health, and wellbeing.

The **sweet, sour, salty, pungent, bitter, and astringent tastes** combine in countless ways to create the incredible diversity of flavors we encounter throughout our lives. Even the same substance can taste different depending on where it is grown or raised, when it is harvested, whether it is stored or preserved, if and how it is cooked or processed, and how fresh or how old it is. Thus, taste can tell us a great deal, not only about what we're ingesting, but also about the physical and energetic qualities we're taking in as a result. Referencing Banyan Botanicals website, "taste is assigned a much deeper significance in Ayurveda than we are accustomed to in the West; it is considered critically important in determining the effect that various foods, spices, therapeutic herbs, and experiences will have on our state of balance – body, mind, and spirit."

Following Ayurvedic principles of incorporating all six taste types into every meal, as the chefs did at the Ashram, my cravings lessened immensely. I still find it amazing how using all six tastes completely changed my prior strong longing for sweets over the year. I occasionally enjoyed a chocolate mousse or a cookie from the Boutique, both made without sugar, but I did not crave them by the second half of the year. They were a "nice to enjoy", not a "need to have" - a very different food experience for me.

The Ashram served lacto-vegetarian food, but I still refrained from dairy, which was easily accommodated by the chefs.

To combat my Vata (wind) imbalances (such as dry skin, constipation, and sleep problems), one third of my daily food intake was cooked root vegetables (mostly beets and carrots, and also sweet potatoes). Root vegetables and tubers are high in fiber, a good source of vitamins A and C, contain anti-cancer antioxidants, and are good for liver cleansing to support overall detox from all my past years of inappropriate eating. I also ate rice, couscous or quinoa - depending on what was served - and the many delicious soups (lentil was among my favorites). I also had oatmeal in the mornings, with cinnamon and almond milk, and often saved the fresh fruit served for a mid day snack.

I enjoyed the freshly baked bread once in awhile, but mostly when it was cinnamon raisin bread - my favorite. Bread was a food I limited, due to its generally high sugar content. Over time, I found I had fewer cravings for the bread with so many other good foods to enjoy. I drank herbal tea with my meals. And during the latter part of the study, KP added ghee (clarified butter with the milk products removed) to my prescribed diet in the evenings, to aid with ease of elimination and to provide fats for normal healthy functioning of the digestive system.

General principles of Ayurveda and my guide, KP, encouraged me to eat my largest meal early in the day. This was an area of struggle for me. The food at the Ashram was a true blessing, and I had noticed that my body needed less food in the evenings. Yet my old habit, of eating my largest and sometimes only meal at night, often had me consuming more food than I needed at the Ashram out of habit. Even natural, healthy foods consumed in quantities that are too large will result in the body having to work hard during the night to digest the food. I didn't realize initially that quantity of food, as well as timing of meals, directly impacted my sleep.

The Interconnectedness of Food and Sleep

My body was used to waking up every 2-3 hours - it was habitual after so many years of doing it. And I had a mind that raced, nonstop. Falling asleep was a nightly battle for me which could easily take an hour. When I did fall asleep, as I mentioned earlier, my body temperature fluctuated - starting out cold and requiring socks most nights and then feeling hot and removing my night clothes, only to again be cold by morning. I also frequently needed to urinate during the night.

My sleep habits were not fun to live with.

However, the diet, along with my prescribed herbs, supplements and teas were all working amazingly well from my perspectives. Doing a nightly massage of my feet with castor oil helped improve sleeping and also improved the dryness of my skin. Another prescriptive - "No reading in bed – lie still, quiet, eyes closed, deep breathing with mantra (can use Om or any spiritual affirmation like 'praise God or praise the lord or thank you for life') until fall asleep. In hot weather, to sleep, lie on right side, block right nostril with finger, long deep breathing through left nostril with calming mantra"

My sleeping patterns weren't consistent by any means, which felt frustrating at times, but I was starting to experience stretches of 5-7 hours of uninterrupted sleep every now and then. Sleeping a solid 5 hours or more felt incredible! I had forgotten how good an uninterrupted night of sleep felt. I knew I wanted more of those nights, and my resolve was strengthened to do what it would take to make that happen.

With the relatively supportive environment of the Ashram, my sleep continued to improve over the year. I tracked my sleep and noted each night's experience in my journal. And I only say "relatively supportive environment" because KP would have preferred that I was in bed sleeping earlier. At the Ashram, I generally was in bed and asleep between 10:30 and 11 pm, after satsang. Rising with the 5:30 am bell or earlier, as I did the first few months, meant that I could get 6-7 hours of sleep - if I succeeded in sleeping all night with no interruptions. While this is normally sufficient for someone who is in balance, and regularly practicing yoga and meditation (both of which are Sattvic, balancing activities that boost energy), I had so many years of sleep deprivation that sleeping 8 - 10 hours would have been preferable to start with. However, I did the best I could, and counted every 5-7 hours of uninterrupted sleep as a huge success.

Fresh and healthy vegetarian/vegan fare did not make me feel heavy and lethargic - not like that comatose feeling I used to get after pizza, wine and ice cream, or even a big Italian pasta meal with seafood, fresh bread and olive oil. But over time I realized that if I had a large dinner, even of the lighter Ashram food, I would wake during the night. It was one of many factors influencing my sleep patterns, and it was difficult to pinpoint any one factor as resulting in a particular effect - but this is one that I really believe made a difference.

Another major factor influencing my sleep patterns was my frequent need to urinate during the night. As a karma yogi at the Ashram, I was living in a tent hut, and waking up to relieve myself meant a rather long walk to the communal toilets. The habit of waking up was so strong that even with having to unzip and re-zip a tent, walk the equivalent of half a block outside and then back again, I still continued for awhile to get up more than once - 12:30 am or 1:00 am and then again around 3:30 - 4:00 am, before finally getting up for the day at 5 or 5:30 am.

You might be wondering why I got up earlier than the 5:30 am bell. It was so difficult for me to take the recommended shower, do my prescribed abhyanga (oil massaged on the body), brush my teeth, and get dressed in time to be in mediation by 6:00 am, as was required, that I had to get up earlier. I was just so slow in the mornings. I now realize this was at least partly because I was exhausted and getting too little good sleep.

Sometimes, though, these late-night trips provided some amusement! One of the funny stories about my middle-of-the-night toilet excursions happened after I had been at the Ashram for two months, in late June. It was a Thursday night, following poor sleep for a few nights in a row due to the heat and humidity. During the day, I had prayed for rain to cool things down. I guess I prayed too hard or too many of us had the same prayer, because we had a huge storm on that Thursday night, with bolts of lightening, thunder and sheets of rain.

Lying in bed that night I thought for sure I'd sleep well, as I was so worn out. And I did sleep pretty soundly until about 2 am, when a really loud clap of thunder woke me. It sounded super close to my tent, and upon waking I could hear the rain pouring all around me. I rolled over and tried to bury my head in my pillow and fall back asleep but, with the rush of water coming from the sky, all I could think about was going to the toilet.

I really tried to block it out. I repeated 'Om' a number of times, which usually calmed me, and I tried concentrating on my breathing. Nothing worked. The urge increased by the second, until I could no longer ignore it. Getting out of bed and unzipping my tent, the force and magnitude of rain became even more obvious, and I could see streaks of lightning flashing in the sky. I had my umbrella ready and put on my soaked black and white flip flops that were sitting on the wooden stoop right outside my tent. As I stepped on the stoop to put on the flip flops, my legs became rain soaked in seconds. I knew there was no way I wanted to walk the distance to the bathroom. I'd either be completely drenched or possibly hit by lightning - I realize now that the lightning strike was a foolish thought, but at 2 am, it's tough to think clearly. I couldn't just go back inside, as the urge was imminent. I hesitated momentarily and decided.

Hiking up my pink nightgown, with my plaid umbrella opened above me, I opted to straddle the boards on the stoop, squat, and relieve myself in the dirt outside my tent - something this city girl has little experience doing. I actually laughed as I did it. It seemed enormously funny to me, and at least I knew that the urine would be washed away with the deluge of rain that continued throughout the night. By the next morning the rain cleared and the air was noticeably cooler.

I chose to share this story as it is another interesting milestone of change for me. Before my year at the Ashram, I would have been mortified and upset by this and would definitely not have shared the story with all of you. If I shared it with close family members, I would have been very embarrassed and sheepish about it. Today I am laughing about it, and I can see the immense humor in the scene. I call that progress for a Pitta dominant perfectionist, who closely guarded her image in public!

SETTLING IN AT THE ASHRAM

Do not brood over your past mistakes and failures as this will only fill your mind with grief, regret and depression. Do not repeat them in the future.

Swami Sivananda

May and June 2015

"The past few weeks have been challenging and still forward motion was ever present. The decision to give away and sell all my furniture came to me rather suddenly, but easily.

It makes me happy to think some of my favorite furnishings are now in the homes of my family and friends. The rest of the items are helping others economically furnish their homes. That was the fun and easy part. Plus, the money I made will help in my savings for Yoga Teacher Trainings and Ayurvedic Practitioner training fees.

What a struggle in scheduling pick ups and getting my life belongings pared down to store at my mom's house! Even with all the purging and donating I'd been doing for months, I was left with 'lots of stuff'.

I was shocked I needed to make three car trips to Mom's, with back seat and trunk of a mid-sized car completely full. Definitely more than the 10 boxes I initially told her I'd be bringing to store. Luckily, Mom was a pretty good sport about it, and Jeff, you wonderful, strong, friend from Landmark - you were a true Godsend to help me move and for loading and unloading the car.

What a time of emotional ups and downs! John's (my son) family move from Chicago just two weeks ago, was sad and joyful at the same time. I was so happy for them and happy I got to babysit quite a bit as they prepared to move. It was a blessing to have the special time with my little grand baby, Vivian, that's for sure. Yet, parting is never easy.

And how fortunate was it that my Jenn's family visited Chicago for 4 days, the week after John, Beatrice and Vivi left. Such joy in those daily visits and quality time playing with, reading to and hanging out together with little grand baby, Aurelia and Jenn and Conrad. Completely unexpected and another true blessing! I loved creating more memories to take with me.

It was also nice to spend time with Mom and (my brother) Steve's family. Their love and support was important to me.

And that special going away party was some Farewell Fiesta, as was the theme! Sandy, Daureen and Colette outdid themselves by transforming my nearly empty place, with decorations and flowers and fabulous food and drinks. It was so nice of the 30 or so people who stopped by during the open house to bid me farewell, share warm hugs, love and give support. It was a fun and happy send-off. I will miss them all.

Then there were the last two days, that had me completely 'out of sorts'.

I was dropping and breaking things, burning myself with the steam of my tea kettle, spilling water as I tried to pour it from my Brita filtered pitcher, with the lid strangely popping off, bumping into the edge of my countertop and landing a nice bruise, and other mishaps throughout the two days.

The goofiest thing I did was thinking I was texting back and forth with someone to set up a meeting for him to come and see my couch for sale, before the final pickup from the Salvation Army. The whole time I thought he was someone that was the boyfriend of a another friend of mine, and when he came to see the couch and I asked him about his 'girlfriend', he looked at me completely puzzled, as he had no idea who I was talking about. It turns out he saw the flier about the furniture on my friend Jeff's company bulletin board. Totally unrelated -

We both laughed at my mixed up mind. I needed yoga.

This morning I felt physically exhausted, having been too excited to sleep much. I was also a bit anxious. Wondering if I would easily get an Uber so early in the morning, I contacted them at 6:15 am, and was in route by 6:22 am. My big suitcase was so heavy, I was grateful that [the driver] Cedric was strong and such a gentleman to happily lift my cases into his trunk. I felt the day started out with good energy with Cedric.

Rather than my original plan of taking the Uber ride to the train, since traffic on the roads was often terrible in the morning, Cedric said that he could get me to O'Hare in 40 minutes. Somehow, I trusted him, and he took me the whole way and right on time - no problem.

What an experience to chat with Cedric, a Gospel singer who leads at the Sunday House of Blues Gospel Brunch, and he has a side business of creating scented oils and incense. He's a talented, jovial man and I was so grateful that he was my ride this morning :)

The next part of the travel was less fun. When I was frazzled and in the midst of chaos, my imbalanced Pitta was raging strong. I was determined to fit everything I needed into 2 suitcases, and with the help of my packing genius friend Daureen, we did it.

Those suggestions of 3 suitcases by others, somehow went in one ear and out the other. The logic of 3 suitcases never registered during the packing phase of the preparations. All I could think about was how hard it would be for me to walk in the airport with three suitcases. I rejected the 3 cases suggestions.

So, due to my stubbornness and inability to think clearly, I ended up paying a $200 overage charge for a suitcase with 67 pounds. The $35 for a third checked bag would have been a much smarter solution. Oh well, next time I'll know.

I was so happy that a man at the Nassau airport offered to help me with my large suitcase, and yet another one came to my rescue when I got dropped off by a taxi at the end of a dock that led to the place I'd catch the boat to Paradise Island and the Ashram.

The taxi driver also shared that it had rained for three days straight and all morning. The weather had just turned. As I entered his cab, it was sunny and in the 70's. Yay!!! I was feeling relief that the travel was over and joy about this new adventure.

I registered, got my tent location, had a delicious dinner and then went to orientation for my karma yoga (selfless service assignment). We were encouraged to skip satsang and get unpacked and settled in. I was glad.

I love my tent space, and especially the attached area with a long writing table that I'm writing on at this moment. I will enjoy writing in this space and feel very happy as I shut down for the night to get some rest.

What a fantastic first day! " (May 1 Journal Entry)

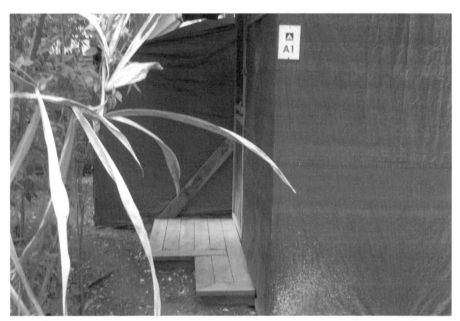

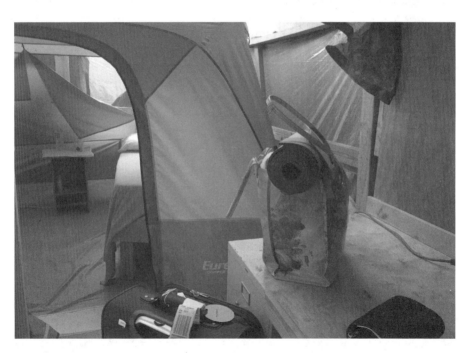

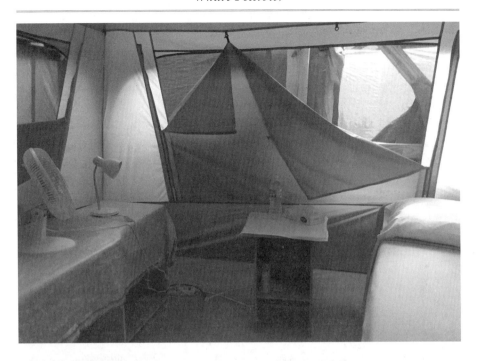

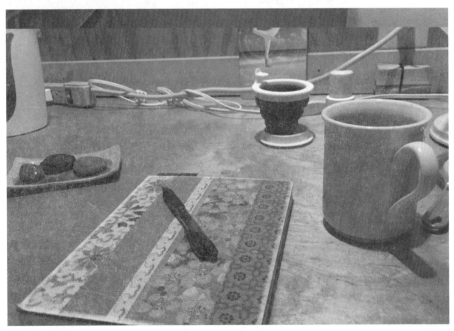

This is one of my longest journal entries, as I had time to settle in before my karma yoga started. The karma yoga residential program at the Ashram is an immersion experience of residential study and yoga, wherein selfless service (karma yoga) is an act of offering our services for the benefit of others, while purifying our hearts and connecting us to the divinity within us and all beings. I understood little about karma yoga when I began, and had no clue how my heart would be purified. I wasn't even sure it needed purifying, and I didn't fully understand what karma yoga or purification meant until many months later. What I did know was that I would contribute 6-7 hours of work each day in exchange for my accommodations, daily yoga classes and satsangs, and the delicious vegetarian food.

I didn't know anyone and, while I was mostly excited, as I sat in my tent hut that first night, the enormity of my decision began to sink in. I had one more day to acclimate and then I would be expected to follow the complete schedule, including my karma yoga duties.

I knew the schedule of the Ashram from the perspective of a guest. The schedule of a karma yogi is quite different. Depending on the duties of the karma yogis, schedules vary. Each karma yogi is required to attend morning staff meeting, one yoga class a day and both morning and evening satsangs. The hours of expected work on top of this are arranged with supervisors, and vary according to where a karma yogi is placed. The 7 - 8 pm Sadhana activities are highly encouraged but not required. Maintaining a Spiritual Diary is required.

5:30 am	-	Wake up bell
6:00 am	-	Satsang (meditation, chanting and lecture)
7:30 am	-	Help clear the platform of cushions and pillows
7:40 am	-	Staff meeting
8:00 am	-	Yoga classes
10:00 am	-	Brunch
6:00 pm	-	Dinner
7:00 pm	-	Chanting of the Bhagavad Gita (sometimes referred to as the Yogi's Bible) or doing Swadhyaya (self study of scriptures)
7:30 pm	-	Community chanting
8:00 pm	-	Satsang (meditation, chanting and lecture or presentation or kirtan music)
10:30 - 11:00 pm	-	ready for bed, Spiritual Diary and lights out

I quickly learned that the 5:30 am wakeup bell required an immediate move into action for me, in order to make the required 6:00 am satsang on time, and it was not easily achieved. Showering is highly advised before meditation, and KP Khalsa also advised abhyanga (self body massage with oil). Having Vata imbalances, the oil massage tended to calm the nervous system and also helped to make me less fidgety in meditation. Because of this extra morning ritual, I considered it a blessing when I woke before the bell, but I never set an alarm the entire year I was at the ashram.

"5:30 rise, shower and get ready for satsang and back to tent to dress - all seemed very rushed" (May 2)

"Woke at 4:45 and took shower and nice not to rush." (May 11)

"Woke at 5:18 am - the perfect time - yay - got a good shower and didn't have to rush - a nice start to the day!" (May 12)

"A Very Good Day - I woke at 4:59 am and showered, trimmed my nails, did abhyanga and got ready for the day. No problem being on time for satsang." (May 24)

"I slept pretty well, considering the heat and humidity. The fan helps a great deal. I woke at 5:25 and managed to shower and get to satsang on time. It helped that I had everything ready from the night before." (June 16)

All the karma yogis were required to be "checked in" to satsang, as it was considered to be a very important part of the study program. Most days I barely got situated on the cushions at the required time, before the initial chanting of 'Om' began. After some guidance and instructions, silent meditation followed for 30 minutes. *Jaya Ganesha* was the opening chant, and then usually another one or two chants were led. Most were in Sanskrit, but we also sang Amazing Grace, The Prayer of St. Francis of Assisi and We are One in the Spirit, all in English. A chant is simply a prayer that is sung, with the main difference to other traditions being that the Yogis sing their chants in a call and response fashion. One person leads and sings a few lines, and then everyone else repeats.

The final part of the satsang was a lecture or teaching from a senior member of ashram staff, or a visiting speaker, that typically lasted until 7:30 am. Afterwards, the platform had to be cleared of cushions and pillows, as it would be used later in the day for yoga classes and workshops. Helping to clear the platform of cushions and pillows comes as a request to the karma yogis and anyone else who wants to help. It always seemed miraculous to me how quickly and efficiently pillows, cushions, and chant books were stacked neatly into the storage cupboard.

Immediately following the platform clearing, karma yogis moved to a different area for the required staff meeting. When the weather was nice, we met in the open-air tennis court area. If it was raining, we met in the covered, open-to-the-sides dining area. Staff meetings always started and ended with prayers. The daily schedule was read out loud, along with yoga teaching assignments, and if any assignments in any of the departments were left unfilled, help was requested. Usually such requests came from the kitchen, who often needed help to serve the meals or unload food deliveries. There was rarely much of a wait before someone volunteered.

Most of the year, there were two yoga classes taught at each time slot - Beginners and Intermediate. When there were not too many guests, during the low season, just one All Levels Class was taught. I usually liked to do a morning yoga class, but it wasn't always possible, and depended on my work for the day.

I have already mentioned that the majority of karma yogis contributed 6-7 hours of selfless service a day. All karma yogis, however, were required to work 7 days a week. This took some getting used to, as I - and most of us - were accustomed to depending on our weekends as 'down time', 'catch-up' time, or 'personal time'. Seven days a week of service was a challenge for me and for most karma yogis. For the first six months, I bounced back and forth between feelings of struggle, frustration, and resentment about having no personal time, and then thinking I was adjusting just fine. I typically entered morning satsang in an annoyed state. Usually when I was exhausted or feeling very stressed, Rukmini would notice and suggest that I take some time off. Once she left the Ashram for six months, I tended to push myself beyond my own limits, but that was part of what I needed to learn. Little by little, the struggles of the schedule lessened, and were much less of an issue for me during the second half of my year. Once in awhile, I entered satsang in a peaceful state of mind.

> *"It's strange how weekends feel no different here than week days. Karma yogis and TTC students have the same work and classes on weekends as during the week." (May 17)*

> *"I'm starting to adjust to the routines here - the early rising, the two meals, my karma yoga work, taking herbs and making teas for the Ayurveda study - it's seeming a little easier.*

> *I enjoy so many of the people here - lots of great energy!" (May 29)*

> *"I never know what day it is, as there are no weekend differences to gauge by." (June 5)*

Swami Vishnudevananda believed that karma yoga should be done everyday, as it is a yoga practice of purification. Working selflessly, without concern for the fruits of the labor, provides us with countless opportunities for self-growth and lessons to be learned. Understanding karma yoga as I now do, one of the most relatable examples I can think of is being a parent of an infant or young child. Caring for your children is selfless service, without any concern about the fruits of your labor. No two days are the same, as far as the duties go, and each day provides a unique opportunity for learning. You don't set your own schedule, and you are 'on' 24/7. Children rarely thank you or give you any kind of recognition for being their parent, and the "job" provides countless opportunities to develop virtues like patience, kindness and generosity.

An interesting early May observation came after two days of rain.

"Both days were filled with lots of rain and dampness - yet the spirits seemed relatively untouched here - even with soaked belongings and sloshing through pools of water it rained so hard - yet everything contin-ued and not in a frantic pace, but rather in the same, calm fashion that life unfolded here on sunny days. Interesting!" "(May 5 and 6)

The first few months were a test of my determination and a period of some major adjustments. Living in a tent hut, when I'd never camped in my life, proved inter-esting. I started out with such confidence, thinking, 'how hard can this be?" Just as with most things, it wasn't really that hard, but it took me some time, some annoyed and frustrated reactions, and some lessons in humility before I learned to manage.

There was a fair amount of rain in May that led to frequent water inside my tent, near the door flap. A pool of water formed inside with each hard rain. Inevitably, I'd step in the puddle first thing in the morning on my way to the shower. I'd grumble a bit and usually remember to avoid it on the way back from the shower. Then after satsang and yoga, I'd diligently mop it up, after borrowing a mop from the housekeeping crew, until the next time. Some of those karma yogis with tents on the ground, though, had their tents and belongings completely flooded, so I felt that a small pool of water wasn't that bad. It took me weeks to figure out that the water seepage was due to an opening where I'd left the tent zipper undone on the bottom of my door flap. I had been struggling to open and close the one main zipper up and down, plus the vent zippers. Most of the time I was doing this in the dark - so I never noticed that there was another zipper to mess with on the bottom of the tent. With what felt like a hectic schedule from morning until bedtime, I just hadn't taken the time to really look and find the problem.

It was an easier problem to solve than the insects, other creatures, heat, and humidity of an island environment. It took time for me to not jump or tense up while brushing my teeth with all sorts of flying and crawling critters hanging out at the bathroom sinks and on the mirrors by the lights. And the walk to the showers

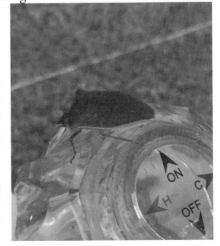

sometimes included gecko lizards and snails and often cats. Eventually, though, I came to realize that the geckos were not seen when the cats were around, and so I rather liked seeing the cats near my tent. Luckily, some evenings were a bit cooler, and I did have a fan. The moving air helped with the heat and also the mosquitoes and insects. Having grown up with air conditioning, I was not used to the heat, especially when sleeping. And, having so little experience with living nestled in nature, many of my journal entries the first few months mentioned my struggles with the weather and also the bites I was getting, especially on my arms, from the typical insects in a tropical island climate.

"...The warmth and moisture of the air feels heavy tonight - and the slight breeze feels lovely. More rain is coming - will be nice for sleep if not a downpour." (May 12)

"Today was particularly warm and humid, and seemed difficult today. My arms and legs are itchy with bug bites...." (May 21)

"..The continual flow of rain. The light breeze barely cooling..." (June 2)

"Very hot and humid today - felt sticky all day long - tough to feel light and cheerful today. The air was oppressive and very little breeze...." (June 10)

"...so grateful for a/c in the office. I can't work in my tent during this hot and humid weather.

I'm really looking forward to going home for Vivi's birthday. My arms are all bit up and look awful. I'm hoping Mom doesn't say much." (June 11)

"I slept pretty well considering the heat and humidity. The fan helped a great deal..." (June 16)

"Weather is still hot and sticky - either I'm getting more used to it or there's a little less humidity as I'm less impacted by it somehow - maybe due to a/c while in the office? (May 20)

"Another busy and hot day. I hardly slept last night due to the heat.... when I worked in the office with a/c it was much easier to breathe and I could think better..." (June 25)

"I prayed for rain to cool the heat of the day..." (June 26)

"Back to hot and humid today...again thankful for a/c in office..." (June 28)

My routine of taking the prescribed herbs and teas required getting used to as well. I didn't have the conveniences of my own kitchen or setting my own schedule. The herbs I had ordered were in bulk size packaging, and I had brought enough for nearly 6 months. I had to figure out where to store them in my tent, and how to find the time and ways to transfer the powders into smaller containers for daily use. I worked with baggies initially, and then tried a few different things before I settled on 1 oz. pill-sized plastic containers I found at a local store.

I was taking quite a few herbs and supplements in different quantities, and had to label the baggies and then eventually the bottles I used. They needed to be small enough that I could carry them in my shoulder bag to go to meals, but that meant refilling quite often. And between the humidity and being shoved carelessly in my bag, the labeling tended to rub off pretty easily. I also had to find the time to get water from the filtered water faucet for teas - which was nowhere near my tent of course - and then make the tea in my own kettle. More time was needed for cleaning out the seeds from the kettle after I drank the tea so that it would be clean for the next batch. Getting some type of routine down for all this was not easy, and there was much trial and error in settling on a system that worked. As it turned out, rarely did the routine last very long, as some change in my day or my accommodations ended up requiring a completely new plan. Lessons in patience and 'letting go of expectations' were often on my path.

Whenever I mentioned to KP about the challenges with taking all the prescriptives in my new environment, he'd inevitably reply "do the best you can". And so, I did.

None of this sounds all that difficult now, as I am writing this to share with you, but initially, as I was learning the Ashram and my job and people's names and the routine and the chants and how to fit in doing laundry, and on and on - it was very challenging and seemed overwhelming.

The yoga classes and satsangs, even with the early morning wake-up required, were supporting me during this time of transition, even though at the time I had no idea that the community energy was helping me as much as it was. The meditation and chanting in satsang were done initially with agitation and then somewhat routinely for me at that time I didn't understand the full impact of the practices until after quite a few months. The evening presenters were often inspiring, and as varied as an expert on quantum physics lecturing on consciousness, a chaplain from Princeton speaking on "Nourishing the Environment", a panel of neuro-scientists dialoguing about conscious, self conscious and empathy/compassion, to Gaura Vani & Kindred Spirit leading lively kirtan chanting for Bhakti Yoga Fest. Each night was an interesting dive into new ways of thinking for me. I had never before considered whether empathy was the enemy of the compassionately conscious self, and yet I found the discussion of the question fascinating. As part of the Neuroscience and Spirituality Symposium in March, a panel including neuro-scientists and professors of religious studies discussed the aforementioned question and other thought-provoking questions. One presenter that I found particularly interesting was Dr. Michael Spezio, PhD. MDiv, affective and social neuroscientist, who was part of the panel. He presented what follows, called The Trolley Problem, as an interesting study in human behavior to ponder.

Scenario 1:

There is a runaway trolley that will kill 4 people unless you pull a switch that kills one person. Would you pull the switch?

Interestingly, in this scenario, the study results revealed that people will readily pull the switch.

Scenario 2:

A fat person can stop the train, if he's pushed off a bridge - he'll be killed, but 4 will be saved. Would you push the fat person off the bridge?

In this scenario, people did not want to directly push the man to save the 4.

Both seemed awful scenarios to me, yet it seemed helpful for me and others to ponder such situations.

I attended the satsangs, and though usually exhausted during the evening presentations, I soaked it all in, albeit with a slightly tired and foggy brain. The yoga classes were my favorite part of each and every day, during the entire year. I always felt renewed after a good yoga class, and in the beginning I needed the energy boosts and calming effects of the yoga poses. You might think I would never choose to miss a yoga class, but as much as I loved them and actually needed them, I did miss classes - too many.

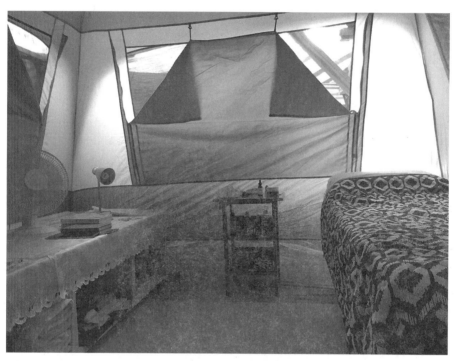

BATTLING WITH MYSELF

An ounce of practice is worth a ton of theory.

Swami Sivananda

July and August 2015

I moved into an air conditioned room on July 1. Automatic joy, right? Not exactly - there was an entire week of little sleep, problems and some revealing lessons that followed.

Space for all the essentials I had brought with me for a year was a necessity for me - at least I thought it was. I had brought with me enough supplies to last a minimum of 6 months and, in some cases, the entire year: things like shampoo and conditioner, soap, abhyanga oils, toothpaste, herbs, clothes for cool and hot seasons, an herb scale, a grinder for seeds, books for reference and to read, extra flip flops and sneakers...the list went on. You may recall that on my initial flight from Chicago, one suitcase had weighed 67 pounds, and the other had weighed in at just under 50 pounds. In my defense, I had no idea what would be available to purchase, and I already knew that the Bahamas were very expensive. So, I brought as much as I could.

> *"Wednesday night, I moved into Om 8 - this was where my journey began when I visited the ashram as a guest in January :) I was so excited to have enough space and this auspicious room.*

Yet, the first night I hardly slept. Om 8 is next to one of the Swami's cottages, and she had high power lights put all around her place. One was directly in line with my windows. They must not have been there in January. My room was lit up even more than it had been in Om 7. I creatively resolved the issue after asking around a bit for fabric or card board to no avail. I used big black trash bags, held to the back of the window curtains with small binder clips - works like a charm and can't tell there's garbage bags on the windows from the inside or the outside. Room is always darkened, but that's ok, as night time sleep is most important to me. Some battles aren't worth fighting. This room will be great!

I also moved into Rukmini's office and am liking the clean, quiet space. I've been getting so much done, and the days are flying by." (July 8)

Om 8 wasn't the first room however. I was first assigned to the air-conditioned room called Om 7, and not being able to sleep due to bright lights , I asked to be moved after one night. My request was granted and I moved all my stuff into Om 1, where there was a much better light situation but where it was so cramped that I was claustrophobic. All my stuff had nowhere to go, and filled so much of the room that it became really distressing for me. So I requested again to be moved.

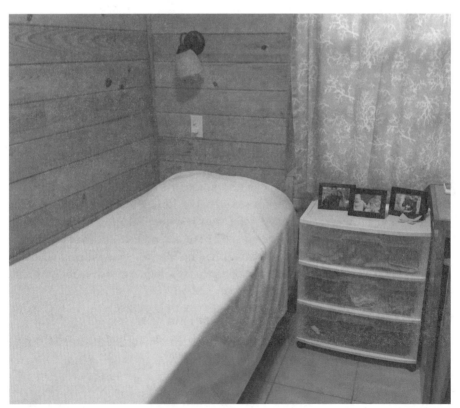

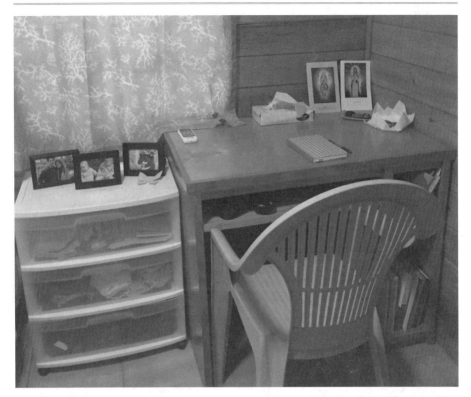

Finally I moved into Om 8 - only to face another light issue! This time, however, as described above, I was able to resolve it, and was much happier with having more space. Also, I felt comfortable in Om 8 as it was the same room I had when I first visited as a guest in January.

While all the back and forth of room changes were frustrating, I was lucky the rooms were close to each other and was so grateful that the Ashram was trying to accommodate me and all my stuff, especially since I would be in this room until the middle of October. It was evident, as I now look back, that my 'letting go of expectations' lessons were not yet learned, although the darkening solution showed me making some progress.

Early July brought with it a big change for me spiritually, as I received mantra initiation and also a new spiritual name. A mantra is a short phrase that praises the holy name of God. It is repeated mentally to help focus and calm the mind during meditation, and brings the devotee closer to the Divine. Many traditional lineages in yoga perform mantra initiation ceremonies by which yogis are "gifted" the specific mantra that they have chosen. Once chosen and initiated, the mantra should not be changed, so it is actually quite a significant commitment . At the Ashram, we were also given the opportunity to receive a Sanskrit spiritual name at the same time. My birth name, Mary, is a holy name in Christianity and respected as such in yoga, but I figured I could use all the spirituality I could get. Most karma yogis who have them use their spiritual names rather than their birth names at the Ashram.

Both the mantra initiation and receiving a spiritual name were completely voluntary, and there was no pressure whatsoever to do either. However, the mantra initiation ceremony and the giving of spiritual names was only done once a month, at the end of the Teacher Training Course (TTC). Since there were no more of these courses scheduled for the summer, I decided to dive right in.

"TTC (teacher training course) graduation was a lively and beautiful occasion. Padmavati is my spiritual name. It is another name of Lakshmi. At first I felt a bit disappointed to not have Lakshmi, as I thought I would receive. I never heard of Padmavati. 'Padma' means lotus and 'vati' means possesses - thus possesses the lotus. Wealth, abundance, generosity and beauty are attributes of Lakshmi and thus Padmavati. I googled and stayed up late trying to find out about my spiritual name." (July 5)

"Rukmini and Swami Hridyananada both sent nice notes about my spiritual name - they made me feel good." (July 6)

"Today, it became official that there will be TTC in November, which is when I will take it! :)" (July 8)

It seemed my flow of good karma continued at the Ashram, as it had been my sincere hope that I could do yoga teacher training in my birthday month of November. I felt blessed by the news, and I was the first person to sign up and pay my registration deposit.

The summer months are quite naturally a slower time in some ways. There are fewer guests and fewer karma yogis at the Ashram. In December, January, and February, it is not unusual to have a total population of around 300-350. It's quite logical that vacationers prefer to get out of their cold climates and come to the Bahamas during the winter, and there is a tremendous energy with all the guests, presenters and students taking teacher training at that time.

During the low season, it's more typical to have a population of around 100. I found that the summer is quieter and quite lovely. The smaller population makes getting to know people a little easier, and there is a closeness among the staff that is not so apparent during high season, when it is so busy that there isn't time to share stories and personal lives like we did in the summer months. The summer is also a time when the senior staff lead more of the lectures in the morning and evening satsangs. Each of the senior, permanent staff are extremely knowledgeable and capable speakers. In their past lives, a couple were lawyers, one was a physical therapist and another a university professor, to name just a few. With this mix of excellent speakers and fewer outside presenters, there is a bit more flexibility in the flow of the satsang schedules. My favorite part of summer satsangs was that the chanting was led by different people, and sometimes karma yogis or guests were asked to lead. It was really nice to have the variety of chants that different people chose, and to experience the support that came to every person who was new and unsure, as they led a chant for the first time. It was a heart-warming experience.

> *"Today was an interesting mix of calm and productive. In the morning satsang, I led a chant - Kali Ma - it is still one of my favorites from the time I arrived, and so I chose it. It felt right.*
>
> *After satsang and yoga, I chatted with a woman guest who said I did a nice job chanting and she said, "you are so relaxed." It was such a strange word to associate with myself. I've never felt nor been called relaxed before. Even when I've gotten massages or nails done, I'm always being reminded to relax, because it just doesn't come naturally to me.*
>
> *This is an interesting change that I will ponder a bit..." (July 11)*

After two whole days of the 'relaxed me' being at the forefront, it was decided that I would take on a new responsibility. I had been assisting Rukmini and learning from her while she was still at the Ashram. By June, I was handling much of the leadership responsibilities of the Communications Team, while Rukmini observed and then counseled me on the ways of the Ashram and alternative approaches. She also continued to meet regularly with me to convey her directions about the overall functioning of the department. I loved working with her, and we made a great team. I was more of a conduit of leadership during that time. I led Rukmini's directions, and I was quite happy doing whatever would help her and the Ashram.

I had known from the start that she wanted me to 'hold down the fort' while she went to Israel for six months, and I had assumed that we would continue to function in much the same way, as it seemed to work so well. What I hadn't anticipated was that, around the same time, the part-time professional Marketing Director would leave her position at the Ashram. I was designated to temporarily fill that role until another permanent professional could be found.

> *"Day was full speed ahead - lots of work with Marketing Director, am transitioning with her, out of her position. Rukmini wants me to fill that role - and while most of it will be familiar and enjoyable, I'm a bit hesitant and want to insure that I don't get dragged into a high stress situation. Maintaining work balance and a filter of love will be the biggest challenges." (July 13)*

I had already been meeting weekly with the Marketing Director, but now the various staff that worked with her would be my direct responsibility. And it was a very busy time. Production of the Fall catalog, plus online uploads of all the programs for the high season were both underway, while posters needed to be created for every presenter and program for the season. These were huge tasks for the teams we had in place.

I also learned that the Marketing staff had not been very stable over the past couple of years. Karma yogis came and went on a regular basis, with some staying for as little as a month, others for three or more, as they did in other departments in the Ashram. Some of them had relevant professional skills, but many did not, and work still needed to be found for them to do. Meanwhile, the professional consultants were all part-time, and worked off-site in various locations. The most senior of them had been working with the Ashram for fewer than 3 years. While all of the professionals were highly skilled, experienced, talented, and dedicated devotees to the Sivananda lineage, not having the whole team on-site made for some interesting communication challenges at times. There was also the reality that they had to get used to a new team leader. The majority of them, having grown tired of the constantly changing staff, preferred to work directly with Rukmini, but this was not feasible given her commitments in Israel.

I told Rukmini I was up for the challenge and that I'd do whatever was needed to help out.

I'd lived through limited resources before, and while this was a completely different set of variables, somehow there was such a sameness about it too. I'd heard a version of all of this in other work environments. Deadlines, personality conflicts, too much work with too little time, tension, misunderstandings.... I anticipated many lessons to be learned in the days and weeks ahead. I was so busy anticipating, in fact, that I missed the first lesson for some time. I felt really good about being able to fill in for the Marketing Director role - and Karma Yoga is not about ego-building, but rather ego-dissolving. Little did I realize how much more difficult this new role would make my efforts to bring balance to my mind, body and spirit.

"My days are consumed with work right now." (July 14, 15 and 16)

"Another day of work filling the hours - no yoga today and still no laundry. My hope for tomorrow is more balance - yoga, laundry and moving my herbs out of the staff room - and maybe a draft of my blog and/or beach time.

I'm working hard to not get pulled back into the stresses of work drama that I've known so well in years' past. There's plenty of personality clashing in this group, and some defensiveness, typical with change. I plan to keep my positive and loving filter intact - not allowing others to drag me into negativity." (July 17)

"These two days were a blur - From the moment I woke to the time I put my head down to sleep at night, my thoughts were work filled. Working on the catalog revisions has thrown me back into the old and familiar

workaholic mode. Helping Rukmini to lead the Communications Team has also been a huge added impact with regard to more emails and transition work. (July 18 and 19)

"Everything I own is dirty - laundry finally got finished after having not one top left to wear that wasn't dirty and sheets needed washing too. So happy to have it done, but I realized I've been missing herbs and not making teas, missing yoga - all a slippery slope to imbalance." (July 19)

"Busy but better paced day - went to yoga." (July 21)

"Woke with strong headache that dissipated with drinking water - think I forgot to drink enough water in the heat yesterday." (July 24)

"Another poor night's sleep and getting up to go to the bathroom in the middle of the night - feels like I'm going backwards with sleep." (July 25)

"My biggest challenge at the moment is from a woman who is the old me magnified 10X - she looks for 'what could possibly go wrong?' all the time. She believes it is for the protection of the Ashram and means well, but she also gets involved in areas that are not her concern and riles others up needlessly. If there is an ember already nearly extinguished, she fans it until it once again flames. And then she alerts others about the pending flame that she continues to fan. She's causing me stress and troubles right now. Oh well - this too shall pass." (July 25)

I came to love and admire this woman very much over the course of the year, but initially, she was truly a royal pain. The good thing was that unknowingly, I had benefitted from all the meditation, chanting, lectures and yoga enough that I recognized she was my mirror, from the first time I met her. My observational skills were improving, and it helped me to have some empathy and understanding of her ways. I also came to see how dealing with me must have really been a challenge for many others along my career path, as I found dealing with her to be a true test of my patience. I wanted her intellectual skills and energies to be put to more positive use. She was a master at asking tough questions that sometimes unearthed significant possible potholes on the path. She also slowed down progress to a standstill, as her continual drilling of questions led to misunderstandings and confrontations that often resulted in tempers flaring or hurt feelings. The repercussions of dealing with all the emotional turmoil caused total chaos at times and complete shutdown at other times. My own 'lightning rod' status had been an issue for me to come to terms with throughout my career. It was so interesting to now be able to observe these personality traits and developed skills in action in someone else. Trying to deal with them in a loving manner was my current challenge. It was a big one, not helped by the fact that the day-to-day stress and missing yoga had been impacting my sleep.

"Busy days of work and meetings. After more than a week of not sleeping well, I finally had a solid 6 hours of sleep - so a good night!" (July 31)

"...a day filled with meetings and an interview and need to get blog done. One month till London and little Aurelia :) " (August 1)

"Meetings, interviews and full day - trying to play catch up in most all areas - work, the Ayurveda study, my family - days are busy and good, but relentless. I keep having thoughts of taking a day off - sleeping in and catching up on my personal things, yet I also have the pull to keep going to satsangs and pushing forward with each day to see What's Possible? Generally my time is pretty happy and I feel good about my contributions, but increasingly I feel tired too." (August 2)

"Today's weekly meeting with Swami Brahmananda brought up patience as a major topic and also balance of work and Sadhana (spiritual practice) through devotion in our karma yoga. Interesting discussion.

Tonight is a big thunderstorm and earlier this afternoon, lightning hit on Ashram property and caused some electrical damage." (August 4)

Stress manifests in each of us in different ways. Since I'd been at the Ashram, my body and mind had the opportunity to ingest healthy and blessed foods daily, plus the benefits of meditation, pranayama breathing exercises, chanting and yoga classes. I also gained immensely from the karma yoga, as it was through the karma yoga that we are faced with lessons to learn and are able to practice virtues. Yet, initially, I didn't realize that the work was providing me with lessons. At the time, I only saw added pressures and duties, which meant more hours and faster work output. I started skipping an occasional yoga class or even a meal, and thought about work all through meditation. I missed going to Bhagavad Gita chanting, even though I really enjoyed it. I substituted karma yoga for other forms of Sadhana, and in my mind I was doing my duty, which I thought was a good thing.

While working, I did get signals from my body to take a break or go to the toilet or rest my eyes. The more I slipped back into the familiar territory of 'work hard no matter what', though, the more I pushed through the aches in my neck or back, the occasional cramp in my leg, or the urge for a nature call. I was used to pushing myself, and there was so much work to do and not enough qualified help. I was not only leading, but also doing the social media posts and some graphic design work to help with posters and a host of other tasks at the Ashram. I kept 'putting up my hand', just as I did as a little girl, saying "I'll do it" or "I can do it." The pace I was once again choosing for myself was bound to manifest in some type of sickness for me. The positive gains of the yoga and other Sadhana practices were overshadowed by the lifelong workaholic syndrome I'd become so used to. Sickness or injury was the only way my body could make me stop and listen.

"I woke with a bug bite or some reaction by my eye - it hurts and is annoying as my sight is partially impaired - still went to yoga and worked all day and fit in laundry - so a full day for sure. Hope I wake up with eye feeling better." (August 5)

"Bad night - up, on and off until 3:30 am, then slept until I heard chanting at 6:45 am. I slept right through the wake up bells - so tired and eye hurt.

Took a quick shower and went to last 1/2 hour of satsang. Was miserable with eye quite swollen and lower eyelid sore. At staff meeting, Minakshi offered to have Nally drop me off at the health clinic. I needed to get relief -

Trip to the clinic was fine. I waited in a clean but crowded room for nearly an hour and a half. There was an intake intern for weight, height, blood pressure and temperature. The doctor checked my eye. My eye is infected - doctor didn't know from what, but prescribed drops to take 3X a day." (August 6)

"...in the waiting room - a woman was on the phone arguing about a check she'd sent 3 months ago and two others were arguing about something else, and the TV had a program with a game show of guessing the star's name associated with a variety of topics from Motorcycle riders to Good cooks, an ambulance could be heard in the background and the phone occasionally rang - it was a chaotic cacophony of noises, and I found myself repeating my mantra. It was so great - I wasn't annoyed with the wait or the people, as I usually would have been. Instead, it felt as though I was detached from all of it while I was there and knew everything going on. Such an interesting experience." (August 6)

"...The day was very busy with work - started the day with 160 emails unread and ended with 54 not yet handled or filed. Finding time for my blog or anything personal is increasingly difficult. There's much work, and I still find it challenging to stop the work and set limits. I'm working on it, and I hope to get some relief once the team gels better and we get some more new people.

My eye is feeling better and the swelling is going down." (August 7)

The doctor at the clinic had said to take it easy and rest. I slept in on August 7 and missed the first hour of satsang, joining in late. Then, you may note with the above journal entry, that I worked on the computer all day long - reading and handling emails no less, even with an infected eye. I said I was working on setting limits, but that was just me deluding myself. I was continuing in exactly the same fashion. I didn't even recognize the work focus as being stressful at all - it all felt so familiar and normal to me. My Rajasic tendencies toward nonstop activity and my Pitta drive to excess were leading the way.

Looking back at my life, I never thought that I was sick very much. Most people, including me, would have said that I was very healthy. Yet, while preparing for this writing, I noticed that I'd been sick quite a few times at the Ashram. Initially, this made no sense to me, as I was eating such a healthy diet, taking herbs and supplements, going to yoga, and meditating and chanting - all good for me and advocated by KP as beneficial in getting to a more balanced state of being. So why was I sick?

It dawned on me that the reason no one thought of me as sick much back home was because I typically continued to work through it. And when I had total breakdowns, I had weekends to just stay in and sleep and rest as much as humanly possible. If I worked long hours all week and partied hearty on one weekend, by the next weekend, I'd have to stay in to recover. When co-workers, friends and family saw me, I was mostly a picture of health, and was considered a strong-willed woman when I worked while under the weather, so to speak. The reality was that I was sick quite a bit.

> *"...I'm still using drops to get rid of the infection on my lower eyelid, but swelling is down and I feel much better. I worked a long day and am getting caught up with work and did some prep work for the Strategic Planning Session later this month." (August 9)*

> *"Time keeps marching on and the days are going by more and more quickly - I'm not stressed out at all, but I feel as though I'm treading water as quickly as I can." (August 11)*

> *"...Lightning struck here - was a huge cracking sound and frightening at first. I was on a work call when the strike hit and the power went out. In less than a minute, the senior staff were knocking on doors and telling us to unplug all electronic devices and to stay indoors - they handled everything with calm and efficiency.*

> *With no internet phones or computer connections for more than 5 hours, the afternoon was free! I wrote my blog and read for 25 minutes and went to the beach for 20 minutes in the ocean and then showered before dinner - wow, what a nice afternoon.*

> *"Lightning strike damaged generator and our meeting space with a/c won't work. Second option also a 'no', as it's being used for a course. Printers are not working and can't print agendas for Strategic Meetings. Ana, the Programming Director, missed her 1st flight, due to a tube of lipstick detaining her at security, and then she missed the second attempted flight when her car broke down. She ended up meeting with us via Skype remotely. Meetings will be cramped in the small office, but*

it will work out. Obstacle after obstacle and intense heat, plus some intense conversations at times - could have dragged me into old ways of annoyance, frustration and some anger - other than one regrettable comment I made, I was able to adapt, adjust and accommodate. I surprised myself." (August 21)

"I worked instead of doing my yoga practice this morning." (August 22)

"I hoped to catch up today...Instead day was filled with email responses - more than 100 through much of the day and finally by 8:30 pm, I was down to 56. I missed meditation and joined when Jaya Ganesha was almost over.

...Maintaining my own personal balance is in direct conflict with how much time I know the job requires." (August 24)

"I missed satsang this morning, as I woke with a headache and knew I needed more sleep. Staying up until after 11 last night wasn't good, and my head is filled with work." (August 25)

"Worked from 8 am - 8 pm, with breaks for meals only - and short ones." (August 27)

It seems obvious to me now that the support of my Sadhana practice would have helped me to be more balanced and much more efficient, but that never dawned on me at the time. I often encouraged friends, family and coaching clients to have balanced lives. Intellectually, I knew the concept. Intuitively, I knew it was the right answer. But I didn't live it myself.

I even complained at the Ashram that part of the problem with my lack of balance was that Sadhana took too much time. I found all the practices to be quite interesting, but didn't 'get' the real benefits of them. I heard the words that were said in lectures, but they didn't really register. I saw benefits from my asana practice, but I didn't comprehend why the other practices needed to take so much time away from my karma yoga. They seemed nice enough to do - the chanting and meditation and pranayama - but they took so much time from "my needed work". The idea of the duty part seemed clear to me and the most important. Still, Rukmini and Swami Brahmananda kept encouraging me to do my Sadhana.

It took me many months - actually most of the year - of reverting back to my old work habits, a couple of bouts with illness, and two infections to finally realize that I was making the same destructive choices again and again. No one at the Ashram ever suggested that I should miss yoga or a meal or be so consumed with work that I could not meditate. It was all me and my mind doing battle against myself and the positive changes that this Ayurvedic-Yogic lifestyle would bring.

I want to confirm my strong belief in discipline, hard work and doing one's assigned duty, whether it is in a karma yoga environment or in a paid, professional environment. An honest day's work for an honest day's pay is as relevant today as it has always been. My work habits though, went way beyond an honest day's work, and I've struggled with the imbalanced, driven nature of being a perfectionist workaholic since I was a little girl. Seeking perfection was the goal, and if it meant re-doing a homework assignment and crumpling up 20 sheets of paper and re-writing it all in order to have an assignment with no errors, then I'd keep redoing it until I was satisfied. My trash basket was often full of these crumpled-up papers. Luckily, today we can save on the paper and merely do revisions with some cut and paste clicks.

Being productive and working to one's capabilities does not have to mean driving oneself to poor health. Balance is the key. I knew the theory, but I struggled with the practice of this simple truism. Not to worry, though. Karma yoga and the Ashram gave me plenty of practice at facing down this demon.

HURRICANES AND STORMS WITHIN

Cultivate peace first in the garden of your heart by removing the weeds of lust, hatred, greed, selfishness, and jealousy.

Then only, you can manifest it externally. Then only, those who come in contact with you, will be benefited by your vibrations of peace and harmony.

Swami Sivananda

September and October 2015

The first hurricane, called Tropical Storm Erica, developed in late August. I had never experienced a hurricane in my life and had no idea what to expect. Initially, I was so busy with work that I didn't even realize there was an impending hurricane threat, despite the news on the internet. Just as with rain storms, everything at the Ashram pretty much continued in the usual calm and orderly fashion, and there really wasn't much going on other than conversation and preparations to protect the windows. The senior staff were very experienced in what needed to get done, and they quietly went about doing it.

"I woke with a headache...Most of the day went pretty well - lots of rain and now talk of a possible hurricane is at hand. We cancelled one of our presenters who was due to fly in tomorrow, as a precautionary measure. Wifi is still working and I continue to inch my way forward to catching up on so many emails and other work..." (August 25)

By the next day, though, it became obvious that hurricane evacuation preparations were taking place. Tropical Storm Erica was building in intensity, and guests were assisted with arranging to return home or to relocate. Some karma yogis were nervous, and texts from home about the hurricane's progress increasingly fueled their nervousness. I felt surprisingly calm.

"Ganesha is leading the hurricane evacuation prepping. He's been through hurricanes quite a few times at the ashram before. He came to dinner drenched in sweat and dirt from carrying large plywood boards to cover all the windows of the ashram - it rained today on and off, and is quite muddy on the grounds." (August 26)

"...Storm is coming - much thunder and lightning during satsang -

We are to evacuate on Saturday morning. The kitchen staff is preparing food to take to the hotel we will go to. I also found out reading a 3 day old email from home that I completely missed last week's blog and didn't even realize it. I'll have to quickly write and send blog before there's no wifi access. " (August 27)

"Storm turned away from us and evacuation was cancelled. The day was a good day of catch up, a little laundry, filling up my herb supplies and writing my blog. With no guests here, and it being the weekend for the off-site consultants, I'm hoping for a slower couple of days.

I went to yoga and Gita chanting tonight. I feel good about today." (August 28)

What I noticed most about the hurricane scenario was the seemingly paradoxical attitude of the senior staff. On the one hand, there was a strong belief and faith that whatever happened would happen, and that the outcome was not up to us. There was no panic, nor any real worry exhibited by the swamis or senior level staff. At the same time, there was a very systematic plan in place to protect the Ashram, staff, and guests. For the yogis, it would be disrespectful and unloving to do any less than the most they could to protect the Ashram. While past karma may have brought the storm, the actions of the present are what would create the karma for the future. The Ashram was their home and a sanctuary for others to learn about and experience yoga. They proceeded in a caring manner throughout the ordeal. It was very interesting to live through and experience.

As quickly as they were put up, boards were taken down and put back in storage, and the next few days were pretty much regular days. Guests started to return and we had a nice size population for the Labor Day weekend in early September. I was happily anticipating my trip to London for my grand baby's 1st birthday!

> *"Tonight I found out I have to move all my stuff into a new room - tomorrow, on the day I am leaving for London - oh well, I'll get it done and somehow, I'm not at all upset by it. I'm moving to another room with a desk :) - a little smaller, but it is still a nice room with a/c. The area of rooms I'm in will be having their termite treatments during the next few weeks. Who knows if I'll have to move again, if my new building also has the treatments? Not keen on lots of moves, but realizing I don't have so much stuff compared to other life moves I've been through. I'm so excited to leave for London - can't wait to see little Aurelia and Jenn and Conrad."* (September 3)

> *"...In the middle of the move, the island experienced a lightning storm hovering right over the ashram - quick dash to the office to unplug all electronics and a directive to stay indoors slowed progress on the move. I desperately needed a shower too and hadn't finished packing for trip. I made it to the boat dock w/4 minutes to send a quick email to Omkari apologizing for not getting back to her due to electrical storm."* (September 4)

As I look back on the day of my sudden move, peppered with a lightning storm and the usual bit of nervousness that comes with any preparation for travel, I can see a big improvement in my calmer attitude. I had been going to yoga classes, as well as satsangs and even Gita (Bhagavad Gita) chanting. My Sadhana was providing the balance I needed to deal with the inevitable unexpected things in life. Unfortunately, I didn't comprehend this at all at the time. I was still clueless about how or why any of the practices worked. I just kept doing them to see "What is Possible?" And unfortunately, often, I put them aside, in favor of doing more work than anyone deemed necessary.

My work emails continually mounted in number, and my vigilant tracking of how many remained unopened or were yet to deal with became an obsession. When I worked in the corporate and government worlds, I had a self-imposed rule about responding to emails within twenty four hours and at the latest, forty eight hours. If I had to stay at work late or get up earlier, I'd do it to meet my own expectations of this response rate. I also had professional full-time staff that could assist when necessary.

With early morning satsangs at the Ashram, and evening satsangs that already ended after my Ayurvedic guide prescribed I should be going to bed, I didn't have more hours in the day to meet the expectation of this prior rule. I also did not have staff to be handling my emails. Somehow, the tension and disappointment that I felt in not responding quickly to people was actually mentally and often physically painful. It is why I sometimes skipped yoga class or delayed nature calls, adding pressure to my bladder and kidney functioning. Besides, I ate my meals in a rush to get back to work, or worked instead of going to Gita chanting. Of course, the more I pushed myself in the work area and avoided the other areas of Ashram life, the more imbalanced I became, and the more mental and physical pain surfaced in my body.

It was a vicious cycle. Instead of working more efficiently and effectively, I was feeling driven, frantic and stressed out. An imbalanced Pitta nature is not a lovely sight. What others saw when they looked at me working in my driven state in front of the computer was anxiety, frustration, annoyance and anger - even if most of those emotions were directed at myself, they were all evident nonetheless. And if others tried to coax me into working less or not worrying about the emails, I rejected their well-intended suggestions. In my mind, I knew better. Once again my body cried out for a stoppage of the insanity, but I didn't really listen. And at this point in the journey, I had no idea how to lead with my heart. I was treading water, using past experience as my life preserver.

"I woke up with no voice and a dry, hoarse cough this morning. I was checked by Dr. Govinda and given a prescription for an antibiotic in case I got worse. Lungs were initially clear. No voice, but I still attended meetings and 'talked' through the chat feature with one team member, who then relayed what I said to others on the conference call. I hope I feel better tomorrow. I'm so tired and my email list grew even though I worked on the computer all day. Frustrating to not be able to get below 100 unread emails - maybe tomorrow." (September 10)

"Rosh Hashanah - nice satsang this morning after missing two days, as per Swami Brahmananda's instructions due to bad cough - I still can't sing. I've been working every day and got emails down to 80 today... Rosh Hashanah celebration was fun and interesting and filled with lots of delicious foods." (September 13)

"Morning meetings and PPT (powerpoint presentation) and then just before dinner I got two venomous and critical emails about the promotion that started today... Reviewing the process and many, many email exchanges confirmed lots of touch points...I missed satsang and worked straight through to 11:45 pm, slept very poorly and awoke tired." (September 15)

"...Emails are still flooding my inbox and not yet under control - less than 100, but just under and need to get it down to 20-25 to be comfortably in control." (September 16)

"A good day and quite a bit accomplished - laundry done and down to about 55 emails, plus a new system that Iswara showed me that may prove helpful. Karma yogis are helping but also requiring my time to keep them busy. Interesting dilemma to need help but not have the time to train the people to help. Things are progressing though and each day is a little better organized - so improving." (September 19)

And when the Ashram work situation wasn't enough pressure to 'break me', I got some outside help from a mix-up with a payment to my electric company back home, alongside an email notice about an unauthorized use of a photo on my blog posts. The payment confusion was easily sorted, and it turned out that the email was a scam, but my reaction to these added pressures was not good. I was still struggling with the extreme side of my intense and driven nature, which always seemed to surface when I was under pressure and was accompanied by frustration, annoyance, anger, disappointment and other unpleasant emotions. When in balance and in moderation, intensity and drive can be productive and good qualities. My daily lessons were about balance, moderation, patience, harmony and equanimity. Still, those long held habits of my life were tough to change.

"...I wonder what past karma these two notices on the same day were from - have no idea if it is this lifetime or a prior one, so not worried about it - but curious." (September 22)

"...I started Positive Thinking course today and first day was ok - pretty introductory, but good to review and the Meditation Room is a nice air conditioned space for the class. The 12-2 timeframe of the class has me scrambling to have enough time for work that needs to get done. It will be a rushed week." (September 23)

"...the course is quite interesting and Iswara is an amazing teacher. Satsangs have been good - uplifting and my main chance for calm and escape from work." (September 24)

"...Catching up on emails and working on Programming issues, plus the time for our Positive Thinking course and a meeting made the day fly by.

To Do for 3 weeks: Going to bed saying "Day by day, in Every Way, I am getting better and better." Also say first thing when wake in the morning. Day 1. " (September 26)

"It seems that I am finding myself in a more agitated state of late - satsangs and yoga are good and positive times, but I must be needing some time off and time for the beach or myself, as I just feel irritated more than usual by people. Mainly my karma yogis on site and one in particular who has a rather laissez faire attitude about work...I'm likely feeling resentful, even though I work so much of my own accord and

because I know what's required to do a good job. And I have some pent up frustration about doing so much. Interesting dilemma - doing my best or choosing more balance - still struggling to find both." (September 29)

Have you ever noticed what anger does to your thinking ability? In a heated argument, for example, have you ever been so angry that you said things you never should have said and usually never would? Or have you been so upset that you can't even come up with the words you want to say to the other person - your mind goes almost numb? Or when you are ranting and raving at the other person, the words don't seem to come out in the order you want them to, and you know you aren't making any sense? I know in the past, I have done all three.

After my year at the Ashram, I experienced and observed in myself, that anger, annoyance and anxiety never made me a better thinker. In fact, emotional wreck would be an appropriate description for me in this frame of mind. I felt hot, flushed and like my insides were churning. I often felt as though I was choking on my own words, as uncontrollable emotions pushed to the surface. As I look back at the internal storms I was trying to navigate, they so clearly show the foolishness of what I was doing. Yet, I couldn't see it. That rajasic Pitta fire of mine was already heated up in the hot and humid environment, and I was making it worse by constantly driving myself to do more and more. It seems obvious now that layers upon layers of unhealthy past practices needed to be peeled back in order to move from constant motion rajas to more relaxed and peaceful sattvic states of being. Thank goodness I was taking all my prescribed herbs and supplements and eating healthy, nutrient rich foods or I could have been an even worse mess.

Around this time, one of our weekly meetings with Swami Brahmananda was particularly revealing and rather humorous. I had noted in my Spiritual Diary that my biggest challenge to deal with that week were those people who sat near me in satsang who didn't want the fan on, while I was so hot. Another one of the karma yogis in our group then complained that the fans that were turned on in satsang were making her miserable, as she was so cold. So try and picture the very real scene that occurred night after night, during the hottest months - the Pittas in the group were visibly sweating and drinking water continually, while the Vatas in the group had long sleeved sweatshirts and sweaters on and big scarves wrapped around them, shivering when the fans were on. And the kind hearted Kaphas, who genuinely care about the feelings and perspectives of others, turned the fans on and off, depending on who looked their way.

It made for some interesting evening satsangs, especially from mid-June until mid-October, when satsangs were held in the smaller Temple rather than on the larger Garden platform. The Temple is a nice, cozy space that is conducive to having smaller numbers of people, and I really liked having the satsangs there, except for the situation with the fans. Swami Brahmananda listened to all of us as we complained, and smiled.

Stormy life at the Ashram continued…

"Ready to launch another campaign and continuing to work as fast as I can to address all the needs and outside emails - down to 86 tonight from a high of 147 earlier today. 86 is still way too many! This evening, we got word that another hurricane is in our vicinity and guests have been asked to leave tomorrow morning. We are on stand-by as to whether we will evacuate tomorrow. A very strange week of red moon, full moon, high waves and wind and now hurricane near - and I can say that most of the pending threat went right by me as I was in the office working away all day every day." (September 30)

"8:30 am meeting and roll call of everyone taken - was frustrated that some people didn't show up until nearly 9 am. At the end of the meeting, I made an impassioned plea for everyone to take meetings more seriously and come when they are supposed to. Then in the afternoon, when we were told another meeting was scheduled for a hurricane update, I was 6 minutes late, and if it hadn't been for Ganesha knocking on my door when he saw the light on and me working away, I would have missed the meeting altogether. I was on the phone with Rukmini - I quickly hung up and joined the meeting. Not Good :(

We are still planning to evacuate tomorrow morning. Boarding was done quickly, in one day with outside laborers called in to help Ganesha. Very quick prep this time and weather feels strange - high waves on the beach and winds really strong at times and then eerily still - " (October 1)

"…We had update of still being in holding pattern and all day we remained boarded up and on alert, but so far no evacuation. Unless storm turns overnight, we should be back to normal soon. Yoga class felt good, as I missed yesterday and have been doing lots of computer work. I ate 2 desserts tonight - not very Ayurvedic, but I did it anyway. They were vegan and delicious!

…The second hurricane was much closer and felt different than the first. We were all still relatively calm, but there were a few breakdowns by karma yogis, showing the strain on people of the past couple of days. I'll be glad when Hurricane Joaquin is past us and no longer a threat." (October 2)

"…The sun came out today and boards came down from the windows. So nice to again have natural light in the office. I got my emails down to 16, working on them from 8 am - 4:00 pm. I did yoga and when I checked, emails were back to 35 - oh well - tomorrow is another day and I'll hope for few emails since it is Sunday." (October 3)

"It was a bright, sunny day today filled with work, blog writing and a nice visit on FaceTime with my family. I also now have a plan for my time away from work while I am in TTC (teacher training course) It's a doable plan with lots of delegation to others. I won't be doing my regular karma yoga duties while I am in TTC, as it is a full time program. Being a paying student at the ashram will be a different experience. I'm really enjoying working with the karma yogi who is assisting me. She's doing great work too. New guests arrived today, and there was a definite energy shift at tonight's satsang - nice to have some new people and happy to be post hurricane threat.

Every day in Every Way, I'm getting better and better." (October 4)

"...Temperatures are quite mild compared to pre-hurricane. My work actually feels like I'm getting caught up, which is nice. I called Mom and talked to her for awhile. She was still worried from the hurricane news and cried when I said good-bye. The media really frightened her and the hurricane was quite real - we were just really lucky and prepared as we could be.

I managed to offend someone today, while trying to give them a pat on the back..." (October 5)

"A day filled with work, controversies and emotional reactions...The funny thing is that Rukmini attributed any and all conflicts to "Mercury Rising" for 3 more days. I have no idea why that has any impact, and initially I found it amusing. Then upon more reflection, this explanation made as much sense as the two grown, successful, professional women in their own rights taking my example personally and completely out of context...Tomorrow will be lots of massaging egos and getting people back on board and out of their funk. Maybe I should wait for three days?" (October 6)

"...way more drama and emotional nonsense than I'd like to be involved in. Today I'm just glad the day is over. It has been a long week. I need a break." (October 8)

"...My foot is not doing too well - may be from bug bites, scratching or skin tear, but it feels painful. I put Neosporin and bandage on it - so hope antiseptic and elevating it clear up the inflammation. I think it will be better if I rest it." (October 9)

"A day filled with stress from work situations, a call that added more stress and much throbbing in my foot. Bhavani's leaving is of great concern, as she does so much for the team and is such a lovely woman... Tonight is the start of Navaratri, 10 days of devotion to the Divine Mother,

3 nights to Durga, 3 nights to Lakshmi and 3 nights to Saraswati. Lots of prasad (blessed food) and beautiful decorations plus candles and chanting - very nice evening satsangs that everyone is enjoying...Email situation has been awful all week, with consultants visiting the ashram and many meetings taking up much of the time....Tuesday, I spent a fair amount of time at the clinic again - Now I have ringworm on my foot, and my idea of a bandage and Neosporin was not a good one. The fungus grew and became even more inflamed with the damp bandage from a couple days of rain and still leaving it on since I didn't have extra bandages - yuck. Lamisil 1%, Benadryl pills and a special shampoos for the affected area are the treatment. What else?" (October 13-16)

There are more journal entries with email counts and mention of my busy work days, but by now, I think you clearly see the picture. What I couldn't see then was just how strong and entrenched our past, learned behaviors and habits become. Through yoga, I wanted to live and learn and lead from my heart, but my head was not having any part of it. After raising children and returning to work, my true emotions were so closely closely guarded that they only made appearances when appropriate or occasionally forced out through anger and times of emotional breakdown. While it sounded like a nice idea, and I genuinely believed I was open to change, the reality is that we like change that is more of a minor tweak than a major shift. Real change is not easy, as it takes time and consistency. My mind fought hard, and the comfort of the familiar was winning the battle. My will was strong and determined to handle the extremes in the same way I'd always handled pressures, deadlines, stress, and criticism - I'd just push down deep my own feelings, plough straight through, head down, and work harder and longer. For most of my life, I had failed to see this approach as unhealthy, and instead had labeled myself as being a leader and an action-oriented woman with a strong work ethic.

In Ayurveda, I learned that toxins are created by emotional factors. Repressed anger as an example, can affect the regions of the gallbladder, bile duct and small intestine. The repression affects pitta, causing inflamed patches on the mucous membranes of the stomach and small intestine. Similarly, fear and anxiety alter the regions of the large intestine. The belly becomes bloated with gas, which accumulates in pockets of the large intestine, causing pain. Often the pain is mistaken as heart or liver problems. Due to the ill effects of repression, Ayurveda recommends that neither emotions nor any bodily urges, such as coughing, sneezing and passing gas, should be repressed.

Repressed emotions create an imbalance which then affects agni, our internal fire of digestion and the body's auto-immune response. In Ayurveda, the root cause of most diseases is low agni, which governs digestion. Digestion refers not only to digestion of food, but also of air and thoughts and knowledge. We digest everything that enters into our body and mind. Repression of emotions mean they still exist in the body, and the longer they are repressed, the more damage they can do.

So many times throughout the year, my efforts to stifle emotions or bodily urges, resulted in eventual breakdown and illness. Ayurveda and yoga recommend that emotions be observed with detachment and then allowed to dissipate. Whether negative or positive energy, it must all eventually flow through and out of the body, or disturbances of the mind and body will occur.

At this point on my journey at the Ashram, there were moments and even hours of progress, but it was slow and not without much struggle and some pain.

> *"...The rest of the day was pretty good. I found out I'll be back in my same tent again, so that's nice news." (October 24)*

> *"6 Days til TTC!..." (October 27)*

As for those weeds of lust, hatred, greed, selfishness, and jealousy - I unknowingly lusted after work; hated myself for not producing even more and faster; greedily desired an empty 'inbox' as the path to peace; selfishly put my mental and physical health at risk by being so out of balance; and was jealous of others who were working less and had time for the beach. I was a perfect candidate for the transformation that we had been told would take place during TTC.

Six Months Milestone

What's Possible?

I usually met with KP monthly via Skype throughout the year. We'd talk and he'd ask me questions about how things were going and what challenges I was having. He sometimes had suggestions for dealing with some of the challenges during the call, but most often, he would just listen intently. Then he would let me know that he'd ruminate on our conversation and send a new prescriptive sheet, outlining what I should take and how much of it and what the herbs or supplements were for. I looked forward to my meetings with KP, but in true form, I also had a couple of occasions where I was so busy with work that I completely forgot to schedule my meeting as I was supposed to do.

My diet continued to be vegan, and 1/3 of my daily food intake was cooked root vegetables -mostly beets and carrots, and also sweet potatoes. As I mentioned earlier in the book, root vegetables are liver cleansing to support overall detox from many years of inappropriate eating. This also supported KP's prescription of a Vata-pacifying diet, with mostly warm cooked foods and minimal cold food or liquid. I continued to eat soups and rice or quinoa, with oatmeal and took fruit in the mornings for a mid day snack. There were also many other amazing creations by our chefs, such as lasagne and shepherd's pie - so delicious!

My dinacharya, sanskrit word for daily routine, was to rise, gather my already laid out clothes, towel and shower caddy and quickly head to the bathrooms. Usually, I placed my things in the shower of my choice and then used the toilets. Sometimes, the toilet stop was first on the agenda. I was supposed to have one cup of hot water, upon rising, on an empty stomach to enkindle my agni (digestive fire). Since I couldn't work out a better way to get the hot water in me while hurrying in the morning to be ready in time for satsang, I basically drank the hot water directly from the shower. Not an elegant solution, but it worked. I also sometimes used my netti pot to clean my nasal passages while in the shower. When I forgot to bring the pot with me, I just cleansed my nostrils by running some water in them and gently exhaling from each nostril separately and using my fingers to remove any remaining phlegm.

After my warm shower and quick towel dry, I did abhyanga with castor oil. None on my feet in the morning - I learned that lesson right away, as oil on the feet is not good for the early morning asana practice - quite slippery. Once dressed, I went to the sink area to use my tongue cleaner and brush my teeth. Then back to my tent to drop off the towel and shower needs. I picked up my prayer scarf and Mobile Meditator (my traveling meditation cushion - can order online from amazon) and then made my way to the satsang gathering, checking in with the karma yoga attendance checker before sitting down on the cushions laid out for meditation.

I continued to drink a mixture of cumin, coriander and fennel seeds as brewed tea in the morning and in the evening immediately after meals, to aid with digestion. Another tea that was prescribed initially was poppy seed tea at bedtime. There was initial success with this. Then in time, the fluids of this tea also resulted in nighttime toilet trips, instead of the deep sleep that was the goal. After some trial and error, the prescription changed to ground poppy seeds that I could eat before bed. I still needed some water to wash the ground seeds down, but less than the tea.

I was still refraining from coffee, caffeinated beverages and alcohol (as was the Ashram's policy) and was eating limited amounts of sweets - mainly special-occasion cakes or occasional afternoon treats from the Boutique.

These are the main Prescriptives I took during the first six months. Dosages often were adjusted based on trial and error and how I felt. A detailed description of each herb and its effects follows at the end of the commentary.

I started with Triphala, Trikatu and Vitamin D3 as I was preparing to start the study.

In April, before I left for the ashram, KP prescribed a full Abhyanga massage with Castor Oil in the morning. Abhyanga is considered an Ayurveda medicine, gently massaging the entire body with warm oil before showering. In my case, I put the oil on after the shower, as the dryness of my skin benefitted from having the oil completely soak in. There is a procedure to follow, starting with legs and feet and working your way up the body, with gentle stroking motions toward the heart It is simple and generally only takes about 5 minutes to do.

I also started on Gokshura and Chyavanprash, plus a poppy seed brewed tea at bedtime. I was not to read in bed, but was supposed to lie quiet and still, breathing deeply with my mantra until asleep. I repeated "Om" as the mantra. To further aid in sleeping in the increasingly hot weather, I was advised to lie on my right side, block the right nostril with my finger and take long deep breaths through the left nostril while repeating in my mind a calming mantra until I fell asleep. KP also prescribed 20 minutes of right nostril breathing, long and deep, in the morning. In Yoga, we learned about the two energies that are twisted and run up the right and the left side of the spine and, uniting, then form the central channel along the spine. The Ida energy, on the left, is the moon energy. It is reflective, calming, cooling. The right is called Pingala and has the energy of the sun: bright, fiery, and awakening. Breathing through the left nostril is a cooling and calming sensation. Breathing through the right nostril is a warming and awakening sensation.

At the end of May, Ashwagandha was added and Tryptophan was also prescribed to aid with sleep. It took me a couple months to locate a source and purchase this in the Bahamas. My experience with Tryptophan was not positive, and I stopped taking it after a short time.

My blood sugar was also originally going to be monitored, and I had brought the equipment to do the testing. Unfortunately, the tent setting and Ashram schedule did not make this testing a viable option. The Ashram did provide a controlled environment, which was helpful for doing a study of living an Ayurvedic-Yogic lifestyle, but it was not a perfect setting in a controlled, laboratory sense. KP and I made adjustments to accommodate for the variables I had to deal with, and I've noted them as well. I tested my blood a few times in the first few weeks and was within a low normal range, which is quite good, so eliminating this testing was not a problem. I ate very little sugar, and though it would have provided additional data, it was not a health need of mine.

In late June, with hotter weather, cool foods were deemed ok but I was still to avoid refrigerator temperature foods or liquids. I occasionally added some salad to my diet. Magnesium glycinate, Shatavari root and Kapi Kacchu were added at this time. Magnesium glycinate needed to be ordered and took a couple months for delivery.

Dosages were adjusted as needed and other changes made according to what I was experiencing while taking the herbs and supplements.

Triphala - a blend of three fruits: alma, bibitaki and haritaki made into powder and mixed together. It is good for all three constitutions and everyone can benefit from the herbal mixture. Besides being a general tonic, it is a light laxative; skin, eye, and liver nourisher; a general detoxifier; and a tonic for the blood, bones, liver, and heart. It enhances production of red blood cells and strengthens the teeth, hair, and nails, as well as improving eyesight and regulating blood sugar. It is one of the strongest rejuvenatives, and an extraordinarily rich source of vitamin C and bioflavonoids. (Caution: it tastes awful - if you ever try it you will need to hold your nose, unless you take capsules).

Castor Oil - The oil comes from the bean of the Evergreen Castor Plant. The bean is deadly poisonous, but the oil is not. Castor oil supports joints, muscles, connective tissue, and skin health. It is used for wounds, trauma and minor pain. It is very effective for organ dysfunction such as an affected liver, menstrual pain, constipation or general abdominal discomfort. It is used to reduce benign masses and swellings, including ovarian cysts, breast cysts, varicose veins, swollen lymph glands, an enlarged liver or spleen, cracked heels and other traumatized tissue. (Caution: it's messy and quite sticky, but it does soak in after a little while. I took this internally, and I also massaged it into my skin daily. It is good for Vata imbalance.)

Trikatu - This three-part mix is composed of ginger root, black pepper, and long pepper ("pipali"), and is used as a mildly warming tonic for enhancing digestion and circulation. This is especially good to fire up the digestive system at meal times. I like the taste of this - it actually spices up food a bit.

Ashwagandha - This is a bitter, astringent, sweet and slightly warming herbal remedy. Ashwaganda is a superb remedy for nervous exhaustion and is considered grounding, while enhancing productivity and endurance. The herb positively impacts general debility, sexual debility, nerve exhaustion, problems of old age, loss of memory, loss of muscle energy, emaciation of children, insomnia, paralysis, multiple sclerosis, weak eyes, skin problems, rheumatism, cough, breathing difficulties, anemia, fatigue, glandular swelling, and infertility. It gives an all-around boost to the system.

Shatavari - In the asparagus family, the herb made from this root is sweet, bitter, cooling and works on all tissues. Shatavari is the main building tonic for women. This herb is used as an effective moisturizer for the membranes of the lungs, digestive tract, and, like other asparagus species, the kidneys and urinary tract. It is an effective rejuvenative to the female reproductive system and the blood, and to build the body.

Vitamin D3 - This is essential for virtually every human body function. I am deficient, most likely from the Midwest location and climate I have lived in all of my life.

Kapi Kacchu - This aids rejuvenation, and increases natural steroid hormones (the good kind). It is good for energy and cognition.

Magnesium Glycinate - This is used to help with nerve support, sleep, and anxiety. Magnesium is actually needed for over 800 reactions in the human body, yet it is the most common nutrient deficiency in America. I took 3 of these every night.

Chyavanprash jam - Traditional Ayurveda jam made in the base of amalaki fruit, a rich source of antioxidants. It has ghee, cane sugar and honey that are carriers for herbs to penetrate deep into the tissues. It is wonderful for rejuvenation, supports proper functioning of the immune system, promotes healthy metabolism and supports healthy lungs and respiration. It tastes good too.

Gokshura - Promotes the healthy flow of urine and supports proper function of the kidneys, bladder and prostate. It tones the male reproductive system, promoting virility, control, and the healthy production of sperm. In women, Gokshura rejuvenates the uterus and helps promote fertility. It calms the nerves, strengthens the body and is balancing for both Vata and Pitta dosha.

While working with me KP teased that he was trying to move the Titanic. With so many years of a fast-paced lifestyle, and a typical American diet of processed foods, plenty of sugary sweets, wine, margaritas, and martinis, so many herbs and supplements were needed to rebuild my cellular health. I looked fine on the outside, but my foundation - inside - was a mess.

Though I wasn't crazy about taking so many prescriptives and looked forward to not having to take so many eventually, at six months it was already quite obvious that what I was doing was working! And a big bonus was that there were no side effects to worry about - only better and better health.

Six months into the study, these are some of the changes that were occurring in my body:

- The whites of my eyes were brighter, and there was no water retention or puffiness visible under my eyes.

- There was generally more pink in my skin tone, which was especially noticeable in my face, nail beds and on the bottoms of my feet.

- My fingernails were pretty much white-spot free; no longer grayish and yellowing, and were less dry.

- The cracks and dry skin on the bottoms of my feet were gradually improving.

- There was hair growth where my hairline was receding, and overall hair growth had increased.

- I was achieving daily normal elimination without coffee.

- I was noticing fewer foul odors when I passed gas.

- A consistent sleep pattern was not established yet, but I was having more nights with longer periods of undisturbed sleep. My longest stretch was 4 weeks in a row of uninterrupted nights and no bathroom trips.

- My ability to sit in a crossed leg position - yogi-style - had improved and the length of time I could sit without moving had increased.

- Breathing during pranayama exercises was much easier. It was initially a struggle, especially holding my breath for any length of time.

- My strength and flexibility had improved. I could hold the headstand, shoulder stand, and crow positions, which were difficult for me to start with, longer and with more steadiness.

- When I went home for the holiday, I noticed my hand strength had increased, as I could again open jars without assistance. It felt great to be gaining strength, instead of losing it steadily as I had been.

- I felt a little calmer and less fidgety.

- My own self-observation skills had improved. I was beginning to see a truer picture, rather than the perfection I wanted to see before.

- My self-acceptance had grown. I was beginning to be able to observe all the many facets of me and was trying not to label them as good or bad, but instead accepting them.

Six Month Milestone - Commentary

By *K P Khalsa*

By six months into this process, we had addressed some minor symptoms and were closing in on the big picture. Since Padmavati was in the vata stage of life, our challenge was to balance vata with a slow, consistent approach that focused on large intestine function, restorative sleep, improving digestion and moisturizing the tissues throughout the body.

Ayurveda has a five-thousand-year history of using unique, sophisticated massage techniques as integrated parts of a total healing system. Ayurveda uses massage therapy as a foundation treatment, not just for musculoskeletal disorders, but for virtually all conditions even the most serious. Depending on the specifics of the treatment, such as the precise oil (often with infused medicinal herbs), the temperature of the treatment room, the depth and intensity of the treatment, the body region worked, and the session length, Ayurvedic massage can treat just about any tissue or function.

All therapy in Ayurveda revolves around the behavior of the body energies. Our goal is to restore balance by offsetting the energetics. Padmavati's symptoms are cold and dry, so our massage strategy was to offset the prevailing energy with warming and moistening techniques and lubrication media.

Ideally, Ayurveda recommends a massage with oil before exercise to increase lubrication in the tissues before the movement. After exercise, when you are cooling down, you could have another massage with a dry, powdered lubricant, such as selected powdered herbs, to absorb the wastes on the skin and stimulate the tissues. The massage should be followed with a shower to remove the herbal powder.

Ayurveda gives special care to selecting oils and other massage media. Each oil is seen as having specific therapeutic properties and is chosen according to the individual client and her relative energy balance at the time.

Oil massage (abhyanga) is performed with much larger quantities of oil than Western styles. This oil is very important to the medicinal aspect of the therapy. The oil is food and medicine and must nourish the tissues properly, so the preparation is carefully chosen. The most common, broadly beneficial oil is sesame, with almond as a second choice. The goal is to get as much medicated oil to penetrate the tissues as possible to pacify the energy being treated. In this case, our target was high vata, so I chose castor oil, the number one vata-reducing remedy in all Ayurveda.

The choice of massage oil depends on the individual's energetics. If the client is metabolically cool, oily, and heavy, with a tendency toward edema, we might use mustard, corn, jojoba, olive, and safflower, which bring balance to this energetic profile. If the client is hot and oily, with a tendency toward inflammation, we could choose between coconut, pumpkin seed, rice bran, safflower, sandalwood, and sunflower, which are cooling. If the client is cold and dry, with a tendency toward stiffness and constipation (sound like anyone we know?), we might use avocado, castor, olive, or wheat germ oils, which are moisturizing and warming. Ayurveda has a trove of sophisticated remedies to offer. With a little study, anyone can bring a whole new dimension to the work of healing.

A note on Castor Oil ...

Grandma might have given you castor oil as a laxative, but Ayurveda recognizes castor as a wonderful panacea for a large number of health concerns. For many, it is a modern day miracle. For people with chronic pain, with aged and damaged tissues, one can soak the body part, such as a foot, in warm castor oil each night for thirty minutes. The relief can be immediate and will often continue to increase each night. Two weeks later, people can be pain-free for the first time in months.

Known as Palma Christi (hand of Christ) in the West, castor oil is pungent, heavy, and sweet, with heating energy. Applied externally, it is analgesic and restores nerve tissue, so it is the main treatment for nerve conditions.

Castor oil is the primary treatment for cold, dry conditions, including constipation and osteoarthritis. The Chinese also use it for joint pain. Following this logic, this special oil is used in the treatment of epilepsy, paralysis, neuralgia, foot neuropathy, sciatica, and many other nervous system disorders. Castor oil supports joint, muscle, connective tissue, and skin health.

The "arnica of Ayurveda", castor oil helps to heal tissue trauma and treats damaged structural and connective tissue and wounds, preventing bruising. It is not designed for acute pain relief, although it is superb for the chronic pain associated with aging and osteoarthritis.

Castor oil works rapidly and effectively to prevent and reverse tissue injury. It is tissue-tightening and helps to stabilize hyper-mobile joints, such as neck subluxations. It reduces benign masses and swellings, including ovarian cysts, breast cysts, varicose veins, swollen lymph glands, enlarged liver or spleen, and lipomas. The gentle application of castor oil to the lactating mother's breasts improves her secretion of milk.

Apply castor oil to large areas of nerve involvement or organ dysfunction, such as an involved leg, or as an abdominal pack for an affected liver, menstrual pain, constipation, or general abdominal discomfort. Use it on burns, bedsores, rashes, skin itch, cracked heels, bruises, sprains, strains, hemorrhoids, anal fissures, torn cuticles, and minor cuts or wounds.

The leaves are poisonous, but they may be steamed and applied externally to relieve pains from bruises, injuries and stiffness, aches and pains, rheumatism, arthritis, lumbago, and bursitis. It can also be applied to infected skin, including warts and fungus, or as a spot treatment for pimples or stretch marks. In Ayurveda, castor oil is used in the treatment of disorders of the nervous system, including epilepsy and paralysis.

Castor oil is extremely messy. Traditionally, it is applied as a moist pack, but compliance becomes a big problem when one is faced with the mess, as Padmavati discovered. A water-soluble gel, castor oil ointment is a convenient alternative. It penetrates completely, leaving no residue.

Use it on specific areas of trauma (anal irritation, etc.). Allow it to remain and soak in as long as possible. Apply it in an abdominal pack for ovarian cysts or liver detoxification. Use it as a breast pack for benign breast cysts. To prevent bruising, apply the castor oil immediately after trauma, allowing it to remain overnight or for several hours.

The energetic characteristics of castor oil are a good match with the typical vata person. The treatment tends to be a little on the slow side, but long-term use can be very effective.

These improvements, while certainly more comfortable for Padmavati, were quite significant from the Ayurvedic perspective. We would like to see a person remain vital to an advanced age. The grim reaper will still win, but how about having great energy, sound sleep, freedom from pain and clear thinking, for decades to come, and then a calm, dignified death? Compare that to the usual many decades long gruesome wind down we see today in aging Americans.

None of the improvements, such as bowel function, sound sleep or grip strength are measurable from common lab tests, and they are so rare that doctors do not even ask about them, but they presage many long years free from pain, confusion and misery from aggravated vata dosha.

Padmavati was already ahead of the game in terms of not having major health crises to deal with, so her transformations were subtler and more internal, but let me assure you that they are very apparent for the person feeling them from the inside. Instead of the relentless march of the clock, and accepting it as typical of old age, how about feeling the clock reversing, and feeling yourself getting younger?

It takes about 5 years for the average American to bring their body energies back into balance, so it take some patience. The results are worth it.

LIGHTING US UP

Illness begins with "i", Wellness begins with "we"

Swami Sivananda

November 2015

The days leading up to taking the Teacher Training Course, referred to as TTC, were much as you might imagine after reading about my workaholic nature thus far. Frantic, driven, determined, and focused all come to mind as ways to describe my days as I prepared to drop the reins of leadership in my karma yoga work for a month. Rukmini was still in Israel and highly engaged with other activities there. I felt and was responsible for the smooth functioning of the Communications Department while she was gone.

In the determined category, I'd reached a milestone just a couple of weeks before the start of TTC. I had always struggled with sitting on the floor, yogi-style, for two hours twice a day during satsangs. I had little trouble with sitting on the floor in the morning , although at times I was still fidgety. Sometimes I could sit still and calm and not have to stretch my legs until after Jaya Ganesha was over - just about an hour in total. It is the longest stretch of time that I have ever been still, even after one year at the Ashram. For me to sit still in any position for an hour is a huge accomplishment. In the evenings, though, I was tired and simply trying to stay awake. Putting extra pressure on my already exhausted body by forcing it to sit on the floor made me really uncomfortable by the end of the evening. So, finally, instead of forcing myself to sit cross-legged in the evenings, I decided to move to a chair as soon as my lower back started giving me warning signs. It was one of my better decisions that actually took care of me.

TTC is another experience altogether, as sitting on the floor in yoga position for the duration of both satsangs was expected. I knew I wanted to succeed in TTC and decided to test the floor sitting out one day in mid-October. Still fidgety, but I happily realized how much stronger I had become, and it didn't seem overwhelmingly difficult to sit on the floor as it had before. From that day on, I managed to sit yogi-style for both satsangs, and began to feel ready to meet the challenges of TTC.

As was the case with quite a few TTC preparations I made, my assumptions were not exactly on target.

> *"1 More Day till TTC :) - the email situation is winding down and I had a couple of good meetings today - If I can connect with Rukmini tomorrow and get just one or two other things taken care of, I should be good to go. I paid some bills finally and still need to send in paperwork for insurance - need to do that soon.*
>
> *Tonight is a special puja (spiritual ceremony) for Swami Prema's birthday - will be nice, I'm sure." (November 3)*
>
> *"TTC start was really a simple transition with an orientation for an hour and the Inauguration in the evening. The ceremony was really nice and we got our uniforms. They called out each of our names and then we gave an offering of flowers and Swami Brahmananda put the powders for purity, knowledge and removal of obstacles on our forehead. We also got our manuals for the course. Everyone had to go and change into one of the sets of our uniforms (white pants and yellow shirts, for purity and knowledge) and then come back to the ceremony. It was as though our group grew into a big bunch of yellow daisies. There was an immediate sense of bonding.*

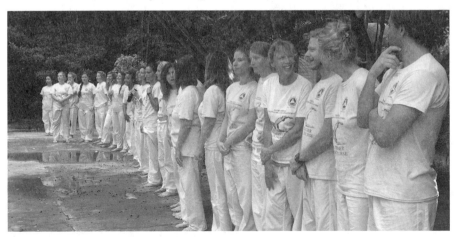

It was also Krishnadas' and Nirmala's birthdays. Nirmala is one of our main Hatha Yoga teachers, along with her husband, Satyadev, and Krishnadas is a senior staff member. It was a special night." (November 4)

"1st full day of classes. It was a good but exhausting day. Adding 4 more hours of sitting in yoga position was really tough for me - harder than I thought, and I'm really feeling it tonight. The classes were interesting and good. I even went to the beach for ten minutes, as Satyadev and Nirmala assigned us to do some beach time :) But now I'm exhausted. I just finished my homework for tomorrow and have to go to satsang - more sitting - argh. I'm hoping my body gets used to this." (November 5)

"The day flew by and no beach time today - really hot in classes. I think my Pitta is up with so much concentrating on classes from early morning until bedtime. I ended up sitting on the bench for part of the Main Lecture. 8 hours of sitting cross legged on the floor is already getting to me, and we just started. I'm also running, it seems, from class to class. The rest of the course is good. The heat and sitting are my two challenges. Tired and sore, but off to satsang - " (November 6)

I went from easy transition to struggling pretty quickly. Instead of the four hours of yogi-style sitting a day that I had planned for, I was having to attempt eight, as we were expected to sit in the same style for the four hours of lectures that we had each day. Some of my classmates struggled even more, having only been used to as little as 15 minutes of sitting cross-legged in a day. And as usual, with me, I was so determined to do well and was enjoying the study part of the course so much that I could practically feel the steam coming out of the top of my head. I was concentrating so hard on every word being said, and my determination heated me up even more on the already hot days. Our uniforms were made of a heavier weight cotton than I had been accustomed to wearing too, so that added to my warmth. I exchanged my size small t-shirts and got large instead, so that there would be more room for air to flow. I'm not sure how much it helped, but it made me feel a little better.

"Woke at 5 am again - so early, but good for being on time and getting shower 11, my preferred shower. I decided to use a chair today for the classes. Meditation wasn't great this evening, but at least I did meditate some before the pain kicked in. Still running - Homework is done." (November 7)

I remembered hearing the lectures over the summer about having preferences and the suffering it inevitably caused. I heard the words, but didn't heed them at this point and didn't even observe that I was exhibiting preferences. My mind was focused on the learning, the homework, and trying to get to everywhere I needed to be on time. Homework wasn't difficult, but it took time as we had to provide a daily summary of the main 2 hour lecture. Plus, we often were assigned to review and practice the yoga pose sequences and learn the benefits, to then teach the next day with our partners or groups.

"Woke at 5:17 and was in plenty of time for the Silent Walk on the Beach - a beautiful start to the day. I filled out the insurance paperwork and am asking for help from my friend back home, Mary Ellen. For some reason, there is no online submission for this health insurance. Afternoon yoga class was our first pairing and actual practice teaching. It isn't as easy as I thought it might be - but I'm sure some practice will help. It's a little tough to tune everyone else out and focus. Homework, satsang and the day will be over - each day goes by so fast." (November 8)

"Happy Birthday to me! and our free day too :) Definitely will get to the beach today...

No beach :(

It was a strange day. Around 3:30 am, I heard something drop on the floor in the office area attached to my tent - Again! I got up to investigate, and saw that a tall partially filled bottle of oil had fallen from about 3-4 inches back on the shelf. The bottle had castor oil in it. It didn't make sense, the bottle was heavy, but I was tired. I made my way down to the bathroom, since I now had the urge, and then returned to sleep and woke at 5:15 am - felt very tired in the morning. The morning satsang was a homa or fire ceremony to remove obstacles and make way for learning for those of us who just started TTC. The ceremony was beautiful, but in the temple, where it was held, the smoke was really potent. Being tired and a bit shook from the night before, I noticed the smoke more and it bothered me more. I could smell the smoke in my hair and clothes, everywhere.

Free day meant that I had time to go to the Nassau clinic and get a refill of the Lamisil for my still persistent ringworm problem on my right foot. After a good yoga class on the beach platform, I had breakfast. Swami Brahmananda stopped by as he had talked to Omkar, who told him about my nightly bottles falling on and off my shelves in the office area. It had been going on for a few nights. I originally thought, since Omkar was always joking around, that he was playing tricks on me to make TTC even tougher. I didn't think it was funny, and announced that comment at dinner one night.

He insisted he wasn't doing anything, and likely he had nothing to do with it. Swami Brahmananda assured me that Omkar was not entering my office space at night, and he further informed me that when he lived in the tent, years ago, there had been rats and it sounded to him that it was a rat knocking things over. There was new construction near my tent, and after all, it was an island. After he left, I really felt awful. I had been able to handle the insects, geckos, snails and other creatures, but Really? Rats? [Side note - the Ashram for a number of years has had treatments regularly and has no rodent problem. This was an unusual circumstance.]

All I could think about was that my birthday morning news was that I had rats in my tent. So, I worked for my hour of karma yoga and made my way to the clinic. I felt sorry for myself and distraught all day. After the clinic trip, I again wiped down my tent with Clorox Sheets, wiping every shelf, hoping to dissuade the critters from coming back. I had just cleaned everything when I moved in only a little more than a week ago, so this added cleaning session was more for my peace of mind than anything else. I did homework and chatted with (daughter)Jenn, (son) John's bunch, and Mom. I didn't tell anyone about my latest troubles. I went back to the office to do some more work, and I planned to go to the ocean, and at 4:40, I finally quit working. As I walked to my tent, I remembered that I'd promised to help two of my TTC classmates with their chanting. Oh well, no beach. Took a super quick shower and felt a bit refreshed on the very hot day.

Helping with the chanting, the two classmates seemed really happy for the help. It made me feel good to watch them improving a little on the chant and almost giddy about being able to pronounce some of the sanskrit words finally. My mood just switched. When I went back to my tent, I banged on the door before I went in, and said "I'm home." hoping to make sure my visitors wouldn't surface with me in the tent. I continued with that ritual every time I entered my tent for days.

Satsang was very nice and a beautiful puja to celebrate Mahasamadhi (self liberation and death) of Swami Vishnudevananda - so it was considered a very auspicious day for a birthday, too. There was a cake for me, candle lighting, gifts and a card - all beautiful and very nice. It ended up a good birthday." (November 9)

Do you remember the 2007 Pixar movie, *Ratatouille*, with the rat for a chef? Well, little Remy, the rat, is what helped me survive the next nights. I kept picturing him in my head, with his big smile and cooking in the restaurant kitchen. It was the only way I could fall asleep, and each day I was really so exhausted from our classes.

"Was wakened at 4:40 am and frightened by something falling into the top of my tent right over my head while sleeping. The tent material

sagged down to within a few feet of my head, or so it seemed. When I shined the flashlight from my phone in the tent, I heard rustling all around outside of the tent and the rustling was moving in circles. As soon as it was quiet, I got up and rushed to the showers. I wanted to get out of there and quick!

Not sure what it was exactly, but Iswara's premise was that a cat fell from the rafters that was chasing the rat(s) and might have even caught them. The day was very hot and I had a tough, long day. I was exhausted by evening satsang and then another night of possible visitors. Eeeeesh." (November 10)

"All was quiet last night and no bottles knocked over either. Long, hot day and lots of homework - again exhausted at the end of the day. Body is feeling sore and tired...We had almond milk at breakfast today - Yay!!!" (November 11)

"All quiet as far as animal visitors. I slept pretty well....Classes were all good and work was pretty good too - I'm pretty removed from it, and it feels good to be so. More practice teaching in pairs today - love it :)

Interesting satsang speaker, Dr. Mark Grossman, an optical doctor, acupuncturist and holistic vision advisor. Key point - Function affects structure of the eyes - 90% of accountants are near sighted, while less than 10% of farmers are near sighted - interesting. Also - eyes hold more tension than other parts of the body." (November 12)

"I didn't even realize it was Friday the 13th until this evening ...Day zoomed by - no more critter visits - perhaps issue is resolved?

We continue to do partner sharing and teaching in asana class - not easy and I still need lots more practice. Homework is taking up what little free time I have - very tired tonight too." (November 13)

I also noticed a very unpleasant smell in my office area that progressively got worse during the day with the heat. I mentioned about the smell, and not being sure if the rats were dead or even gone, to Swami Brahmananda. He said if I wanted to move temporarily to a different tent, I could do so. Chatting during brunch with another karma yogi friend, Omkari, and moaning a fair amount about how I didn't need all this emotional turmoil besides trying to get through the intensity of TTC. I was questioning whether I should move now and noted that it would be a pain to find the time to do that too. I was in one of those states of unclear, rambling thinking. Omkari listened and said little other than, "why don't you just Face the Rat?" I thought about it for a bit and then I decided to do just that. I stayed put, determined not to let the rat push me out of my tent and disrupt my TTC.

The foul odor was there for a few more days, and then it just went away - and never returned. Neither did any other un-invited visitors resurface, and I stayed in that tent for another 6 months.

However, that was not quite the end of my nocturnal disturbances.

> *"Woke at 1:30 am and thought I heard a movie. I thought Iswara, my neighbor, was watching a late night movie on his computer. I was knocking on the side of my tent like a wall and calling to him to put on his headphones. After 3 attempts that failed to quiet the noise, I decided to go to the toilet. When I returned, I still heard the noise and called into the night "Iswara, put on your headphones". Of course, none of this made any sense, as no one was watching a movie, but rather the party boats were raging on until 2:30 am from what I was told during the day. Usually, I didn't hear the party boats in the bay, and Iswara wears earplugs I think - so quite the comical scene." (November 15)*

I think my mind was still edgy from the rat visitations. But the experience did have its positive side, as it showed how much my hearing was improving in my left ear. That ear had been nearly deaf before, and when I first arrived I couldn't even hear the party boats if I was lying on my right side.

In the meantime, TTC continued. The teachings that we were gifted with, each and every day, were rich and thought-provoking and voluminous in the sheer amount of material. Each sentence was a lesson in itself. Learning the Sanskrit terms and about the four paths of yoga, the eight limbs of yoga, the seven Chakras, the seven Stages of Jnana or Bhoomikas, the three bodies and three levels of the mind, as well as yoga anatomy, the karma law of cause and effect, and Samsara, or the wheel of birth and death, to name some of the content, was daunting for even the best students among our group. Each topic was fascinating to me. I hadn't been in intense learning like this since college, and even then, I rarely had more than two or three classes in one day. We were immersed in classwork from morning till night, six days a week, for twenty-eight days.

Everyone had warned me that it was an intense experience, and it was. And although I struggled, as did everyone, I loved it. Each lecture was a treasure that I tried to imprint on my mind. Swami Brahmananda taught as though the words came directly to us from Swami Sivananda, the yogi saint who the Ashram is named for. Graduating from the Sivananda TTC, we each become part of the lineage, and inherited thousands of years of teachings passed down from gurus to disciples to students. It's not easy to explain, but being part of an ancient lineage felt amazing to me. I knew that when I would beach yoga, it would not be teaching my lessons, but the lessons of classical yogis from the ancient past. I would be the receptacle and deliverer of the teachings in the purest sense. It was and is a great honor, privilege, and responsibility to stay true to the classical teachings.

I wrote volumes of notes for classes, and the manual we were given was about 3 inches thick. With all that writing throughout the day, I did not get a chance to write much additional about the teachings in my journal. So, much of what I share next is a summary of my class notes. I chose a couple of concepts to share, and hope you find them as fascinating as I do.

Karma yoga is one of the four paths of yoga, and I had been doing karma yoga daily as a contribution to the Ashram since I arrived in May. When I took the TTC training, I was no longer a karma yogi but a student. However, each TTC student is assigned one hour of karma yoga service to be done daily, even on our free day. Karma yoga is the path of action, duty and service. It is sometimes considered the entry path of yoga, to help ready the body, mind and spirit for the other paths. It is also considered a path of purification. Karma yoga is not volunteering in the Western sense of the word, but should be performed selflessly and without thoughts of the fruit, or results of the work. And when you think about it, money is not the only fruit we get from work.

Karma yoga is not something you put up on your FaceBook page to show the good deeds you did, in hopes of your friends and followers clicking "Like". It is also not a duty that you do, so that you can feel pride and self-worth by doing the duty better than others. In listening to Swami Brahmananda lecture about karma yoga, I knew that while I wasn't focused on praise or the sense of accomplishment as I worked, it was indeed what I was seeking. I was sincerely offering my help to the Ashram - that part was pure - but I also wanted to do the 'best' job of anyone on the team. My ego was in control and pushing me in search of that feeling I got when I was 'best' or 'perfect'. I wanted to please my supervisor and satisfy my own expectations for myself.

Yogis teach a lot about discipline and doing everything in a quality manner. There is nothing 'half-way' or sloppy about the yogis. Doing things well and correctly and with care is how we should do everything, but not for the praise or the boosted ego, and not because we are 'pleasers' or because someone is watching. It is more about doing things the right way because we should want to do things the right way, or to the best of our ability, as a matter of principle. Descriptions of behaviors and right actions can be found in the ancient texts, and those scriptures are still followed today. For example, the yamas (ethics) and niyamas (spiritual observances) are much like the Christian Ten Commandments.

The five yamas, or self regulating behaviors, relate to relationships and the outer world:

- Ahimsa: nonviolence

- Satya: truthfulness

- Asteya: non-stealing

- Brahmacharya: non-excess (often interpreted as celibacy, but married couples and consenting adults are yogis too - celibacy as we think of it is for those on a strict spiritual path, similar to a path of priesthood)

- Aparigraha: non-possessiveness, non-greed.

The five niyamas, or personal practices, relate to our inner world:

- Saucha: purity

- Santosha: contentment

- Tapas: self-discipline, training your senses

- Swadhyaya: self-study, inner exploration

- Ishvara Pranidhana: surrender to God

Giving and receiving thanks and praise are certainly practiced often by yogis, but true karma yoga would mean not expecting the praise or the thanks. It is a fine line of distinction, but a really interesting one. Doing things well in the course of duty and service should also not harm our physical or mental well-being. My understanding of "selfless" was skewed by my family and cultural bias. I assumed being selfless meant caring about anyone else but me, or at least, that I should come last - just as a new mother would place her baby's primal needs ahead of her own need of sleep (new parents are excellent examples of karma yoga).

Yet the yogis teach that this same mother needs to follow the principle of ahimsa - a basic tenet of yoga that essentially requires us to do no or little harm to any life - and happily accept help when needed, in order to maintain her own strength. What I hadn't really mastered in my life was the 'doing no harm to ourselves' part. That was and continues to be a difficult and important lesson for me.

The word 'karma' comes up quite often in my writing, and I do find this concept appealing. Yogis say that we all suffer in life, and it is a matter of how equipped we are to deal with the suffering. Our karma bank from the past is like the 'wild cards' in board games, giving us those challenges, gifts and blessings without our having any notice or control over which 'wild card' we get. The most simple explanation of karma is to think of it as results of past thoughts and actions that we live out in the present. Yogis believe that karma can be from this lifetime or past lifetimes, and we don't have any way of knowing which it's from. It is quite different from fate though. While we do not have control over past karma, nor when and how the karma will come to us to be experienced, we do have control over how we react to it and thus we have free will in the creation of future karma. Yogis believe we experience both the Laws of Karma and free will.

Say that we find a $20 bill on the floor at the grocery store as we wait in line to pay. There are a couple of people in front of you, and the lady from the next register line had just reached over to grab a magazine from the rack in front of you. The $20 is only seen by you, and as you bend down to pick it up, you start to think about your good fortune. You have some options of what to do with this 'found money'. You can quietly put it in your pocket and think to yourself, 'ahh, good karma'. You can also ask those around you if any of them lost a $20 bill. In the first scenario, the $20 may indeed have been good karma from the past, and you are now the benefactor of an extra $20. Is it a good decision to quietly put it in your pocket? Not really, because now, since you didn't do the ethically right thing and ask if anyone else had lost the money, you just created bad karma for the future. In the second scenario, if you discovered that someone in line lost the money and you give them back the $20, you have just created more good karma - and really you aren't any poorer for it, as it wasn't yours to begin with. If no one claims the $20, then when you keep the money, you have become $20 richer and have still created good karma for the future.

The teachings about karma also help to shed light on some things that have been puzzling to me for many years. It explains why some 9-or-10 year olds are musical geniuses, or gifted artists or great intellects. Mozart may have been developing his musical skills in dozens of other lifetimes. It also explains why some really distressing things happen to some really nice people. Now, I like to think that their next lifetimes will be so much better if they handle the bad karma well. It may sound harsh to our Western way of thinking, but yogis would say that any bad actions (misfortune or bad luck, we might say in the West) that we experience today are due to similar bad actions that we did to others or ourselves in the past. Those who are poor may have been rich and stingy, not helping others in past lives, and so they are now living out the karma of poverty. Generous actions do not require money. Helping someone who has dropped something, or letting someone else get in front of you in line when they are in a bind, or helping a handicapped person get across the street, are all ways of being generous and giving. And for those of us who are able to help others with our financial abundance, not only does the generosity help those less fortunate or those just needing a little help, but it also creates good karma for our future and insures that we will continue to have that abundance.

I also like the comfort of knowing that every good action and every good thought will always produce good karma, even when at times, it seems otherwise. Bad karma can never come from good actions or thoughts. So, when you don't 'get the job' or 'get the guy' or 'get the raise', it isn't that you've done something wrong. You might have done everything right and been creating good karma for the future. The result of today is always based on past karma ripening in the present, rather than what we are doing right now. It's a rather freeing idea, when we can remember to think of it.

At first I questioned this premise, as we all know of people who have done some pretty bad things, and yet they were successful or had gained fame and fortune or powerful positions. Yogis would say that the success, fortune or high level positions were all the results of past good karma. The people, no matter how awful they may seem now, must have done good in the past. Unfortunately, the negative behaviors of today, like preying on those less fortunate or wielding power as a threat, will all end up producing bad karma for the future for them - either in this lifetime or in future lifetimes.

It also made me think about the cause and effect that I'd grown up with of hard work yielding success. Yogis would agree about discipline and hard work resulting in good karma, but only for the future and only to the extent that ahimsa and moderation were followed. If it were true that hard work yielded success or the desired outcome, then hard work should always result in such success. Yet, we all know of instances when hard work did not result in a successful outcome. Hard work therefore is not the cause of the success. Yogis teach that past good karma causes success experienced today.

Just as Buddha teaches about the "Middle Way", Swami Sivananda wrote these simple words of wisdom that he encouraged his fellow yogis to follow.

Eat a little, drink a little

Talk a little, sleep a little

Mix a little, move a little

Serve a little, sing a little

Work a little, rest a little

Study a little, worship a little

Do Asana a little, Pranayama a little

Reflect a little, meditate a little

Do Japa a little, do Kirtan a little

Write Mantra a little, have Satsang a little

Serve, Love, Give, Purify, Meditate, Realize

Be good, Do good; Be kind, Be compassionate

Enquire 'Who Am I?', Know Thyself and Be Free.

The more I practiced, the easier each day became for me. I tried to be less attached to my actions, and focused on doing my best at any given moment, rather than pushing myself beyond reasonable limits and thus actually creating bad karma. It's still a lesson in progress though. I have had so many years of being the other way, that I cannot expect to change my long-held habits overnight or even in a year.

The yogis teach that what we need to do to insure that our future has abundance and love is to focus on God, give to others, and to love each day. We create our own good karma and create our own futures along with it. Sounds easy enough, right? But in our universe, there are no absolutes. If you do some action, it may be good in one corner of the world and bad in another. The idea is to do the maximum amount of good and minimum amount of bad. The fact that we are born in a human body means that we have mixed amounts of good and bad karma. I'm working on creating as much good karma as I possibly can!

In TTC, besides the lectures on yoga philosophy and the scriptures, we had twice daily yoga instruction on asanas and on how to teach the postures. The classes on how to teach yoga were packed full of information and practical experience. We learned to teach beginners and all-levels classes, as well as adaptive classes for children, pregnant women and those with physical limitations requiring alternative postures and approaches. We practiced with partners and in groups, and led the whole class in Surya Namaskar (sun salutations). We were expected to use the proper terms in Sanskrit and English. We taught with thunder and rain as the backdrop, and we taught with cool breezes, heat and sunshine. We taught with the party boats passing by along the bay, loud speakers and blaring music. Each and every day we learned more and practiced more. No matter the external elements, we continued to practice and learned to teach.

Anatomy was a very challenging class for me. I'd watched the TV show Gray's Anatomy, but other than that, I had no background in this subject. College biology class taught me little about the human anatomy, but it was the closest class I had to draw from - and it wasn't much help, considering I'd taken it about 40 years ago. And the TTC anatomy class was a beast for me. Even though Krishna Das was an expert in the subject, adding more long terms to my list of 'need to know vocabulary' was problematic. While the words were English, they might as well have been Sanskrit in some cases, and learning the systems of the body and how they worked was not easy. In the condensed timeframe of our course, Anatomy seemed quite difficult to me.

Then the time came for the exam.

> *"Our review class was a bubble burst - WAY more information than I expected to have to know for this test. I'm much less excited about the test now - tomorrow will need to be about serious studying - at least there is a study day" (November 29)*

An unexpected experience occurred for me the day before our final exam. It was a day that would be spent studying all day, and it was a time of heightened nervousness for me and all my classmates. We had covered so much material. Like many of my classmates I chose the morning yoga class, in hopes of clearing any of the mental cobwebs and opening my mind for the volumes of information I would be reviewing throughout the day. During the seated forward bend (paschimottanasana in Sanskrit), a favorite pose of mine, I went into a meditative state quite easily and was rather dreamily saying my mantra when I saw Swami Sivananda in a seated yoga posture. He was only there for a second or two, but he was clearly present and calmly smiling at me. This vision felt quite profound.

I'd been doing poses in a meditative fashion for a few months by this time, and had on occasion seen different colors, sometimes eyes and even a few faces of people I didn't know. But I couldn't make it happen, not in the poses nor during meditation, and more often than not I didn't see anything at all. I have not seen Swami Sivananda again since that one time. At the time I wasn't sure what to make of it, and even questioned if I had somehow purposely put him in my mind. I think my doubt about the validity of this vision is why I didn't even write about it in my journal. Today, I am convinced, he was letting me know I'd do just fine on the test.

Though I paid close attention in every class and did all the homework, I hadn't taken a long written exam (over three hours) in many, many years. I had been struggling with the Sanskrit terms the most, and some of them just would not register in my mind. I had been grateful throughout the TTC that I had at least been hearing and learning some of the prayers and chants during the six prior months that I was a karma yogi. It seemed my mind had needed all that time to loosen up a bit and warm up to the new language. Words like tanumanasa and pararthabhavana don't really have any easy correlation to English, and there were many of these words that were equally difficult for this Western-brained American to learn. Yet we were told that there would be about 100 Sanskrit terms that we should study and know.

One of my biggest lessons that I took from TTC involved the exam. I studied hard the day before, reviewed my notes on my own and also reviewed some with classmates and senior level teacher, Iswara. I had the body systems down solid, and I knew the Sanskrit posture names, benefits, all of the class sequences and descriptions, the opening prayer, and about 85 or 90 of the Sanskrit words, but the last ones just were not making it into my head no matter how hard I tried. I kept mixing them up and confusing myself more.

My brain actually felt like it hurt, but that of course was more from the stress I was putting on myself, trying to know everything, than from my brain actually physically being in pain.

> *"Not a good night's sleep - study day today - yoga and did 2 hours of karma yoga and then studied for 7 hours. Iswara helped tremendously by quizzing me before dinner. He has such an amazing mind and memory - a fascinating being. It was beyond nice of him to drop everything else and work with me for an hour or so - I needed it. I still can't get the Bhoomikas!*

...Even though I feel certain that I'll pass, I still am anxious and feel less prepared than I've ever been for an exam. Not that I haven't learned a lot, but I know for certain that I don't know some of the answers. I've always entered exams before, thinking I could get 100%. Not this time - time to study more, just was not possible." (November 30)

"I woke at 4:30 and stayed up - took a long shower and went to satsang early. I chose to do pranayama breathing and meditate, rather than study more. Enough was enough! I realized full well that there were answers I would get wrong or leave blank, and that was going to have to be ok. This would not have been ok with me in the past. It's not that I got a perfect score on every test I took in my lifetime, but I believed I could get a perfect score going into every test in the past. This time I knew I would not get a perfect score, and I just had to be ok with it.

We had a short satsang, a light breakfast and then took the test on the Garden West Platform. We were told to bring a food tray to write on and pens - nothing else would be allowed on the platform. Luckily they decided it was ok to bring our own cushion if we wanted to, and I placed mine behind my back as I sat in a chair. 6 or 7 of us sat in chairs, while the rest were on the floor, yogi style. We were separated and monitored by at least 2 teachers at all times. Paper was given to us and tests were handed out after instructions were given. We had 3 1/2 hours to complete the questions..." (December 1)

To not divulge test questions for future yoga teachers in progress, I will merely share that indeed there was a question about the seven Bhoomikas, and I couldn't fully answer it.

"...I worked on the test, using all the time given, minus about 3 minutes. Only 3 other students were still working when I turned in my exam. The relief I felt was immense, and I was certain I passed. I had some blanks and likely one or two wrong answers where I just guessed. Guessing Sanskrit names isn't really a good idea :)

All of my classmates felt the same sense of relief, and most of us were amazed at just how much information we had learned. Seeing it all written out on sheet after sheet of the exam, made it really evident. It was a good feeling. It really didn't matter that I didn't get them all right.

...The evening graduation was a puja (spiritual ceremony or ritual) and then each of our names were read, and we received our diplomas. After the main ceremony, we gave our teachers gifts of flowers, chocolate bars, hand written notes by each student on cards and a special gift for our main asana teachers, Nirmala and Satyadev. We painted a mandala

that could be hung up at their yoga studio in Colombia, designed by our 18 year old classmate, Lorel. We each painted a portion of it, so it was a true group gift.

...It was a really nice night and happy occasion. I'm officially now able to teach!!!!

After 10:30 pm, I left to make my way to bed - having gotten up so early, and after the tension from the exam, I am really exhausted." (December 1)

The course went beyond my expectations, and I'm not sure how, but we each came out on the other side as changed people. There were days when we felt like we were being tossed and turned in a washing machine, cleansing our bodies as well as our minds and hearts. We came to see life differently, and we felt differently too. We actually sensed our hearts opening, shared in the oneness and had glimmers of understanding of a kinder, gentler, happier and more peaceful world.

I still had many unresolved questions, as TTC isn't an end point, but rather a beginning journey to a new way of life. It felt as though our teachers lighted the path for us to follow.

Some students took the TTC for their own self-improvement and to deepen their practice, while others of us were interested in possibly teaching. I was sure that after TTC, I wanted to teach and share the blessings of a healthy body, the joy of pranayama breathing, and the love that radiated out of me when I practiced yoga.

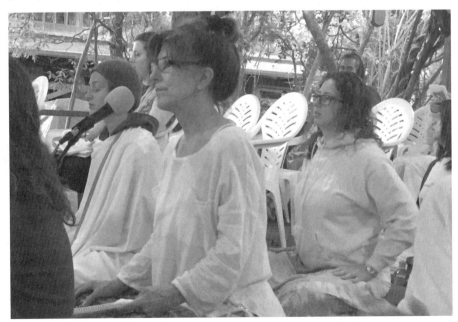

SAINT MAKERS

Be Tolerant.

Behold the unity of all faiths, cults, creeds and religions.

Respect the views, opinions and sentiments of all.

Swami Sivananda

December 2015 & January 2016

December and January are prime time, high season at the Ashram. The population of staff, karma yogis, students and guests swells to 350 on some days and rarely goes lower than 300 throughout these months. It's a time when everyone loves being at the Ashram to enjoy the beautiful weather and amazing programs! Each day is filled with wonder and joy. It's also lots of hard work and some tension is inevitable. December at the Ashram displays a true unity in diversity, as presenters, teachers, speakers, guests and karma yogis from all around the world come together and join in the festivities.

Those of us doing karma yoga continued as usual with our daily work, only now there was much more of it with so many extra guests needing attention. We were often called upon to help with extra duties, such as helping to serve at meals, or cutting up fruit to be blessed and passed out after satsang (Prasad). None of these extra duties were difficult, but the sheer volume of people just meant a little more work for everyone.

"Exhausted but pushed through for 7 hours of office work - very productive and catching up after month away for TTC. Herb supply is low and I am only taking 1/2 of what I'm supposed to, trying to stretch until I get more supplies." (December 2)

"Another 7 hour workday today and very busy - feeling more tired today. Was kind of negative even after yoga today - Omkari suggested I get to bed early. Very helpful I think" (December 3)

"Woke early and felt pretty good throughout the day, but noticed I was a bit grouchy - not like me. Am on top of the work situation, so that is good - something is not right though. More staff arriving soon." (December 4)

"Looking forward to Ayurveda massage treatment - Shirodhara, hot oil massage - my body needs it. Maheshwari is my therapist and was wonderful. She asked whether I'd taken some time off after the intensity of TTC, which I hadn't. Her assessment of my body was that I had severe exhaustion. She recommended I take some time off.

It was easier said than done with so many things yet to do. After a shower, I worked another 5 hours. I was yawning all through satsang." (December 5)

"...Little things matter - like new lightbulbs in the office and a visit from Parvati, who was excited to show me a beautiful, interesting tree and its blossoms. The flowers on this tree bloom only for 1 day and then are gone. She showed me the tree and encouraged me to watch for one of the blooms opening at around noon tomorrow. I know she's trying to get me out of the office for a break, and she's been bringing me fruit for the afternoons to keep up my energy too. I am grateful for both.

Tonight I ate with the presenters in the Swami Vishnu house - was very nice and conversation was good. It was very peaceful too. There are between 10 and 25 diners on any given night in the Vishnu House, but compared to the 300+ people eating in the regular dining areas, it is extremely peaceful.

I found the Sikh researcher and his wife to be quite interesting. He teaches and does research at Harvard and specializes in sleep disorders and the psychophysiological science underlying the benefits of yoga practice. His presentation should be quite enlightening." (December 7)

"Interesting and stressful day - rained pretty much all day and everything feels damp. Our Creative Director, photographer and yogi who will be photographed for the catalog, all arrived today. 4 other new karma yogis for marketing team also recently arrived. At the moment, things feel chaotic. I met with everyone and spent a fair amount of time with the Creative Director. The photographer added the stress of the day, as she began with demands and refusal of the use of her equipment, if her demands weren't met. She's truly a challenging woman and a beautiful photographer - so talented and yet so demanding. She also is not feeling well. Not a good start for the photo shoot -

Meal times are fascinating in the Vishnu House. With Father Meninger, a Catholic monk who is a real character, plus his two traveling companions, lawyers nonetheless, the conversation about the Big Bang Theory and the Trinity Comparisons to Brahman, Vishnu and Siva were lively - especially add in the two Sikhs and the newly arrived kirtan chanting group from Milwaukee, and of course the ashram swamis, and TTC teachers - What a mix and such fun and interesting people!" (December 9)

Having the privilege of eating with the guest speakers was a daily treat. The speakers were so far out of my mainstream existence that the exposure to and interaction with them was quite enlightening. Father William Meninger, for example, based at St. Benedict's Monastery in Colorado, was 84 and walked with the assistance of a cane. His traveling companions helped him to get around, assisted with his personal needs and with his preparations for his presentations, which were spectacular. He was warm, intelligent, funny and very quick witted. He loved to bring up thought provoking conversations, and the Christian Trinity Comparison to the Hindu God forms of Brahma, Vishnu and Siva was one such conversation. His main point was to note the similarities in the foundations of the Christian religion and the Hindu religion. In Christianity, the Trinity are comprised of the Father, Son and Holy Spirit - all representations of God. In the Hindu faith, Brahma is the creator, Vishnu is the protector and Siva is the destroyer of evil - all manifestations of God. The conversation highlighted that the ancient Christian Mystics described God and spirituality in ways that reflected the same basic principles as in the Hindu religion and also Yoga. Each week, the group was different, and I met Shaman healers, a Buddhist Lama, Jewish Rabbis, a Muslim Sufi minister, a PhD professor of Computational Physics, a Vastu Shastra expert (similar to Feng Shui) and Qigong Masters to name just a few.

My karma yoga also continued to deliver lessons, albeit in a subtler way. People went to the Ashram for all sorts of reasons, and were working through all sorts of issues - physical, emotional and spiritual. As we all know, our issues travel with us wherever we go, if we let them. Without the Western cultural veils of office decorum, political correctness, or even job qualifications most of the time, the situations in our daily karma yoga work settings were much more powerful and blatant - definitely an 'in your face' experience, seven days a week.

'Saint makers' are commonly talked about among the karma yogis. During our weekly Sadhana meetings with Swami Brahmananda, there were often questions about dealing with others who were making our lives miserable. The annoying person, the co-worker who agitates or doesn't pull their weight, the habitual complainers - all of these labels are bundled into one, and yogis call them "saint makers". According to yogis, we are each "saints in the making", so to speak, as we learn and grow spiritually. We also are "saint makers" for others when we annoy them, frustrate them, and drive them crazy.

Realizing our true nature requires experiencing ourselves and observing our behaviors, reactions, and thoughts. Meditation provides us with a way to observe our thoughts, while karma yoga provides us with the opportunity to bring our true natures more and more to the surface. It also brings up the emotional "junk" we all carry around. If there is no one to annoy and agitate us, then how can we realize that we are impatient and work on the virtue of patience? If everyone is a top performer and produces work to excellent standards, then how can we recognize what pushes our buttons and stirs anger and frustration in us, so we can learn to be kind, understanding and less judgmental? If no one ever complains, then how would we learn to discern, listen with compassion and go within for our peace and joy, instead of relying on others to share their happiness?

According to yogis, each person that evokes some reaction in us is an opportunity to either detach from our reactions and move on, or to do what we usually do and let our reactions take over. Along with those reactions is usually struggle through all the emotions and suffering that go with attachment. (And detachment, by the way, does not mean disinterest or not caring. It simply means standing back and observing, rather than participating in the drama). Needless to say, for me, the photographer was one of my 'saint makers'. From the day she arrived, there were issues.

> *"Rained out this morning's photo shoot attempts. I went to Anjaneya's staff class this morning, and it was quite good. This afternoon, the photographer showed up with her equipment, and I prayed for good photos. I'm still trying to figure out what work to have new people do. Little by little, every day in every way, I'm getting better and better. :)" (December 10)*

> *"A new task on the "need immediately" list. There's a sudden push for the Foundation to have a website and donation capabilities. No one, other than me, knows much about websites.*

Photo shoots were minimally successful, in part due to rain. I'm not certain how to use Ahimsa when I have to relay negative feedback to staff. Staff issues are the stress of the moment - so much of the work is rather loosely defined and few people have similar work ethics to mine. Without specifically assigned tasks, they are aimless and I don't seem to have enough time to get the tasks on my own plate done, yet alone provide all the guidance and training that is needed by those I work with. Today, I feel totally work stressed." (December 11)

You might have noticed that my obsession with email counts had subsided. After TTC, I was determined that I wouldn't let emails get the best of me every day, as they had been doing. But this didn't mean that I completely changed my workaholic ways. The many new lessons that I learned in TTC had me rising up with a lovely view of the sky, only to be let down hard to the ground with a thud - sometimes all on the same day, and other times with successive days of downs before rising up again. Life felt much like a seesaw, and it seemed that many 'saint makers' were on my path.

"Sun is shining today - a good day for photography. Much else is happening at the same time, including a video for an ATTC promotion.

I assisted in Krishnadas' yoga class this morning on the Bay West Platform. Two of us were assisting, so it was pretty easy - a good first assist.

The day went by fast and I made some progress on the Foundation Website too. I even ordered Christmas gifts online for the girls (grand daughters) :)" (December 12)

"We are in the Bahamas at an Ashram Yoga Retreat, nightly light- ing candles for Chanukah and singing a few Jewish prayers after our meditation and singing the Opening Prayer of Yoga - with pictures of deities of the Hindu tradition adorning the walls of the Temple, alongside Jesus, Mary and Muhammad - with everyone, including a PhD Sikh from Harvard and an 80 year old Catholic monk making offerings of flower petals in the puja (spiritual ceremony) that is led by an Indian Vedic Priest - and the Catholic monk, along with his two accompanying lawyer devotees participating in the chanting which is led by a kirtan group who came from Milwaukee.

*I am living what Swami Vishnudevananda (the founder of the Bahamas Ashram Yoga Retreat) hoped would bring true peace to the world - **Unity in Diversity**, and it is incredible!" (from BestYOU blog posting, December 14, 2015)*

"Photographer has been sick and in her tent for three days. Who knows when I will see the photos she's taken. Good day - busy and went by fast - lights adorn the ashram and Christmas Trees make for a festive mood - weather is beautiful, in the 80's and sunny - really nice!" (December 15)

"Another quick day - hair turned out great at place Bhagavati suggested. I feel good about going home soon - won't be any 'looking ragged' comments, as I look pretty great!

The realization that I will be home soon has set in, and I'm really looking forward to it.

A couple big projects to wrap up before next week - the Foundation Website and the Ashram Holiday eCard to send to all Sivananda Centers worldwide, plus another Communications Team Update and Madhavi replacement search - hoping it will all get done :)" (December 16)

"Meetings and work on the Foundation Website filled this day, plus the afternoon puja. We are nearing completion of the site, and I created letterhead, plus worked on copy and design of an email to be sent to appeal to people for end of year donations. Omkari got the Paypal working, and all but two pages of the site are ready. Sri Devi Sharon was a huge help with the logo and formatting the pages. Tomorrow will be the official launch of the site - no yoga today, too busy - not good." (December 17)

"Worked all morning on the website and graphics for the site. 3:00 pm the email was sent out and website is officially announced! Some corrections were needed almost immediately, but they were quickly fixed and hoping donations will start coming in. Rukmini seems pleased and others have commented positively. The ashram has wanted a Foundation and a vehicle for donations for many years. This year, both became a reality.

Perhaps, this is the real reason I learned how to create a website with Weebly - might have been for the ashram, all along - not sure.

Tonight's satsang was Karnamarita Dasi - an amazing vocalist, chanting classical Indian ragas. It was a fun satsang, except that I was miserable and hot, not near a fan turned on and no breeze at all." (December 18)

"As easy as yesterday was, today seemed stressful and long. I didn't get to do yoga class today, as it was the anniversary of Bhagavad Gita. We chanted the entire Gita - 2 and 1/2 hours long - 18 Discourses (chapters) led by our priest, Krishnan Namboodri.

It poured tonight during satsang, and it was tough to hear concert, but Karnamarita just kept on chanting. The email backlog is again frustrating me. I'm tired of being so far behind." (December 20)

According to Ayurveda, Pitta body types, like mine, are physically of medium build, well proportioned, with medium strength and medium endurance. The basic caution for a Pitta type is to lead a moderate and pure lifestyle. Pitta types respond badly to impure food, polluted air and water, alcohol and cigarettes, and especially to toxic emotions - hostility, hatred, intolerance, and jealousy. Quoting Dr. Deepak Chopra, M.D., "If there is an Ayurvedic type who exhibits the Type A behavior that cardiologists warn against, it would be the imbalanced Pitta-Vata, with Vata-Pitta not far behind."

As I mentioned earlier, my constitution is Pitta with many Vata imbalances. I'm also in the Vata stage of life. And while I have a very strong work ethic, my basic constitution is not the strongest of the three types. Pitta has the strongest drive and is the most intense, but the physical capacity to match is not Pitta's strong suit. My secondary Vata tendencies, with Vata being the most fragile physically and mentally of the doshas, compounded the issues that I often faced. It is Kapha types that have the solidly built, strong physiques that excel in endurance and stamina, and are the most grounded and steady of the three doshas. In balance, Kapha types can live long, healthy and contented lives. We all have some of each of the three doshas in us, but my Kapha tendencies are much less than my Pitta or Vata characteristics. I failed to recognize this particular point about myself over and over again. Before I knew anything about Ayurveda and Pitta tendencies, I equated my intense drive, willingness to work and desire to succeed with a strong work ethic, which in my household was demonstrated by a great capacity to do work. My mother, who was my first and best teacher, has strong Kapha tendencies and Pitta characteristics. She has always been able to do an inordinate amount of work, and continued to be employed until she was 84. She still does physical work in maintaining her own home.

I'd read, with great interest, Deepak Chopra's book *Perfect Health* and a few other books on Ayurveda by KP Khalsa and Dr. Vasant Lad, along with dozens of KP's articles before I started my yearlong study at the Ashram. Yet, until I began writing this book and reliving the journal passages, it hadn't sunk in that I was never going to have the same stamina or capacity as my mother. It didn't mean I lacked a strong work ethic or that I wasn't a hard worker. If I pushed myself to run Marathons, I could, just as I pushed myself to work longer hours and harder than everyone else. I was quite accomplished at driving myself into imbalance.

Because I can, it doesn't mean that I should.

Again quoting Dr. Deepak Chopra's book, *Perfect Health*, "...Pittas tend to go out of balance by pushing themselves to extremes. On the assumption that they can eat anything, they abuse their strong digestion by overeating or forgetting about nutrition. Instead of being natural high achievers, they can become driving, impatient, demanding and tense. Pitta dosha controls the intellect and endows Pitta types with a sense of orderliness. Out of balance, they become fixated on order and annoyingly perfectionist..." That about sums it up...........I was annoyingly perfectionist.

"Laundry, yoga, working on design of Christmas Card for the ashram and generally trying to keep up with meetings with staff on and off-site. January promotion is needing attention Links to fundraising site connecting ashram site and Foundation site is done and video taping commotion is handled. A busy day -" (December 21)

"Leaving for home today...moved things to the other office, as Rukmini arrives from Israel later today. Trying to not think about sharing that other office with 4 or 5 people - maybe will work from tent - not today's issue.

...I'm very excited to see everyone at home and a little nervous too. I'm also looking forward to being at the ashram for the New Year, and know it will be fun to return here." (December 22)

"It was nice to sleep in a dry and comfortable bed... Mom seems happy I'm here..." (December 23)

My holidays and visit home were really nice. It was the year for both of my children's families to spend Christmas with us in Chicago. It was great to see my brother's family and especially spend time with my two grand babies, who brought lots of energy, laughter, warmth, love, noise and chaos to the holiday gatherings. It was a really beautiful Christmas!

If you are wondering whether I kept up my yoga practices (Sadhana) - yes, I did. I meditated, did pranayama breathing exercises and yoga asanas every morning, starting before the sun rose. I found it funny getting up in the morning to the sounds of my mom watching TV instead of the Ashram bell. She is a very early riser, and her TV programs are her constant, daily companions. It took some getting used to, especially to ignore the sounds of the TV when I was meditating, but I did the best I could and was happy that at least I was consistently doing the practice. Mom was pleased that I generally joined her downstairs for breakfast by 7:00 or 7:30 am. My prior self would have slept until 8:30 or 9 on vacation. My late waking used to annoy my mother to no end, as she generally gets up by 5 or 5:30 am.

"Uber driver came 15 minutes early - such a nice guy and helped with my bags too...

Got all my emails caught up since I sat at the airport until 3:00 - was supposed to be flying at 10:40 am...guess who was on the boat back to the ashram with me? The photographer had been to the clinic to get more meds, as she is still sick. She said she uploaded some of the photos, working from her tent. I told her I hoped she'd feel better soon and said thank you for the photos. We spoke no further...

I've unpacked and am ready for bed - though I'm happy to be back, I already miss having my own bathroom attached to my room LOL" *(December 29)*

"Woke early 4:00ish and went back to sleep until 5:08 am - was at satsang early - beach walk :) It was a beautiful day today - weather in the 80's and sunny.

...struggling a bit with a sore left hip - hoping yoga classes will help... Day went by fast, with 3 meetings and an interview with a new possible karma yogi. I'm only so-so on her from the first meeting, not sure why, but something in me isn't convinced she's a good fit. I'm still thinking on this more.

Satsang with Bahai faith leader is on agenda for tonight - am tired, but hope I'll enjoy satsang." *(December 30)*

The interesting thing about this karma yogi that I interviewed is that she did end up joining our team. She also was one of the best karma yogis I worked with during the entire year. She was a true joy to have on the team. Perhaps, without the support of the satsangs at the ashram, my critical and judgmental tendencies had resurfaced after my trip home. Or maybe I was just feeling negative that day. Whatever the reason, I was searching for the 'what's not right' in the interview, instead of leading from my heart and seeing all the good. But hitting a pause button had become a fairly regular practice for me when I felt indecisive, and this was a great step forward. When I didn't assume I had the control and the answers all the time, I received some wonderful surprises.

"New Year's Eve with Gaura Vani

A day of meetings and work that made it go by quickly. TTC gradua-tion at 4:00 shortened the workday, which was nice. Tonight's dinner, followed by Gita and then satsang will be good!

...not sure why, but I am a bit on the low side - might be because my left hip is still sore - better but still hurts. I'm not looking forward to more sitting on the floor. I may choose a chair after meditation. (December 31)

"I managed to stay sitting on the floor and the celebration went on until 1:30 in the morning. It was a fun and full evening of singing, dancing,

pujas and a parade after midnight, all around the ashram following the priest-made mandala that was carried by 4 men.

Our wakeup bell was at 6:30 am and I slept like a log for the 5 hours. I couldn't believe it was already time to get up, when it was 6:30.

I was a few minutes late to satsang after a shower, but it was a good satsang.

More meetings and trying to figure out what to have the karma yogis do - the current challenge. I have little office space and people who need to be using computers, plus some are not very good at seeing things that need to be done, on their own.

I'm tired today, even with my own yoga practice this morning and the advanced class in the afternoon. I hope my hip feels better tomorrow - not ideal right now." (January 1)

"...much stress over karma yogis on site - who does what and works where - 2 small offices with 9 people makes for challenges." (January 3)

"Past two days I've been assisting and demonstrating for Rukmini, who is teaching Essentials 1 Class. So great, and I've enjoyed it, but there is some controversy over who was informed and who should have been informed first. Such a strange dynamic to have power struggles here. A culture of discipline and beautiful philosophy that often morphs into ego issues.

Late night - after 11 pm in bed." (January 4)

"A frazzled day - seems like the team has so many needs, and I am so busy that it's hard to meet their needs. I'm loving assistant teaching with Rukmini!

Hard rains all day and night - everything feels damp." (January 6)

"Just an 'off' day in many ways - my throat is starting to hurt too.

Teaching was great, but rest of the day was just OK and challenging with no yoga. I opened and closed with prayers the Joan Borysenko workshops. Great attendance, with 100 people in her workshops." (January 7)

The next few days of posts have mentions of the fabulous Tao Porchon Lynch, who at the time was a 97 years young, beautiful woman who can command an audience with her stories, still sits in Lotus position (I'm not even close to doing it) , and is the oldest yoga teacher alive in the Guinness Book of World Records. In her past, she was also part of the Hollywood set as an actress and couture model. Tao also helped people escape from the Nazis as a French Resistance Fighter. Her life experience list is long and fascinating. She is alive and well.

> *"...Tao arrived wearing 3 inch high heels, beautiful clothing and jewelry, wearing makeup and a smile that warmed all within her sight. Her escort Terri co-authored, with her mother, Tao's autobiography..." (January 8)*

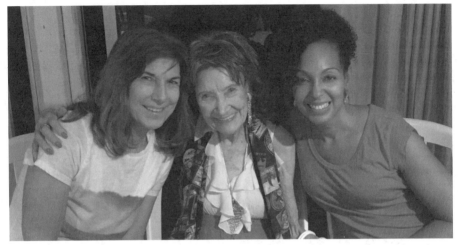

Me, Tao Porchon Lynch & Dr. Terri Kennedy

> *"Tonight Tao speaks again, and she taught us yoga today while sitting in lotus. Incredible! Young and old alike are flocking around her throughout the day. She has time for all of them and has amazing stamina and such joyful peace about her. I've enjoyed eating meals with her and feeling her calm." (January 9)*

> *"...I took Tao's yoga class - so inspirational - and her mind is as sharp as her body is flexible...I bought her autobiography, and she graciously signed it for me. What a woman!" (January 10)*

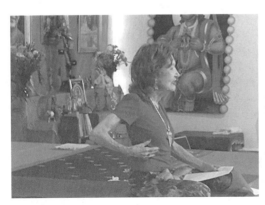 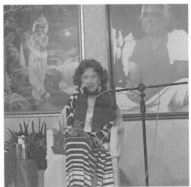

You may have already guessed that my entries were also filled with comments about being sick and continuing frustration with the personnel issues. Did you see it coming this time? My body gave me the signal of a sore hip after the delayed travel day and no yoga, and even continued to give me the signal when my mind considered not sitting on the floor for the New Year's Eve celebratory night. Did I listen and take my own counsel of sitting in a chair? No. With not resting the hip, not getting enough sleep, the stresses of the daily work at hand and choosing to push myself and do advanced yoga, along with one day missing yoga altogether, the sickness was inevitable. The one positive thing I did do was to start taking high concentrations of the Vitamin C that Swami Brahmananda had recommended. At first I balked, but then I listened, and my symptoms lessened until I was soon feeling better. But once again, I hadn't learned the lesson.

> *"Teaching again today :) Rainy off and on - weather not so great, but it is much milder than January back home.*
>
> *...As soon as I manage to resolve the day's issues - from battles over Tripods to not having enough keys for the offices to bruised egos and people basically struggling in too close of quarters - then add in my supervisor's additional 'asks' and people she's added, such as the ATTC student who will join our already unmanageable group. We don't have enough space for the people we have and I have little time to guide their work, but somehow we keep figuring it out. No yoga today." (January 12)*
>
> *"An angry start to the day as one of the newly placed karma yogis spewed anger toward me in a very disturbing fashion. My helping her to be on the team may have been unwise. And I wonder about my own karma and how I've reacted to authority in the past - since karma is a reflection of my own past actions. I've no idea how or why she has become such an angry person, but I do know that I do not have interest in putting up with her attitude, nor her tantrums. I will do my best to remain non attached and continue to include her in a kind way on the team - but it may not be easy.*
>
> *Who knows what happens next, but I will surely find out as it unfolds. Biggest value add of the day was to ask the Vishnu kitchen staff to make my coriander, cumin fennel (CCF) tea for me, and they said Yes! I'll again start having the tea that I stopped making." (January 15)*

The 'saint makers' abounded for me at this time. Occasionally, one 'saint maker' came at me with tremendous force, but just as often, numerous 'saint makers' were in my vicinity at the same time. The small issues became magnified because of the number of them. These added stressors are what we all need to be equipped to handle, and my prior approach of restraining until I strongly reacted, and then begging forgiveness, was not the way I wanted to continue.

I'd become more accustomed to my schedule of taking herbs and supplements, and restarting the tea was a positive for the health side of things. As I continued to explore "What's Possible?", it became more and more evident to me that Yoga and Ayurveda provided pathways for much more than physical health. The mental and spiritual gains were equally significant. I'd not realized before to what degree my habits were ingrained. Nor did I fully grasp the scope of these habits. Intellectually, I knew many of my habits were not healthy nor joy producing, and knew that the strength it would take to replace these habits would be immense. Especially difficult would be those regarding my judgmental nature and intensity in work situations. This was perhaps partly why I had resisted major change, opting for small, incremental changes throughout my life - often superficial - and basically I remained the same.

The yogis teach that detachment helps in dealing with such struggles. I had used mental restraint and repression of my feelings as my way of handling stressful people and situations in the past. Keep smiling, stay positive and bury the negative. That is not what is meant by detachment. To develop the capacity to allow whatever external situation shows up, positive or negative, to not affect your internal state of well being - that is what yogis mean by detachment. My way of restraint and repression would work for a while, until the build up of emotion became too much. Then I would react with resentment, anger, frustration, or a combination of all three.

The "saint makers" lessons kept challenging me and inching me further along. I was increasingly seeing the folly in reacting to others, either immediately or after some time of restraint. I was also improving in actually noticing my own reactions in my mind. The lessening of intensity, not only of my reactions but even of my thoughts, was an interesting development. I am totally convinced that each of these changes were the result of the healthy lifestyle I was living, the medicinal herbs I was taking, and the spiritual energetic support of the Sadhana. It was as though I was building a new me from the inside and tearing down the old me from the outside at the same time, and crazy at is sounds, I could feel the construction taking place.

"My days are filled with work and handling staff issues - from tears to arguments to anger to laziness and pettiness and childish behavior - oh and being stubborn should be on the list too - all have been present with the on-site karma yogis these past few days.

Taking the Essentials 2 Course with Rukmini teaching has been quite positive, and the morning yoga plus lectures are great!

Weather has changed and now it is cool, in the 60's at night. I don't have much warm to wear, so it has felt like a cold week to me.

I taught my 1st Staff Class - yay!!! It was great to teach again and get the 1st class past me - always a bit more nerve wracking. I made many mistakes but recovered from them pretty well. There were 10 people on the Vishnu Platform taking the class - full class. I teach again on Monday, so more practice!" (January 20)

"No journaling past couple of days - been tired and going to bed right after satsang. I've worked after dinner until satsang starts, so no time for writing it seems - just so busy here. I've been struggling with hundreds of emails again, especially after taking the Essentials Course and with the HR side of the job taking so much time - peaked at 320 unread on one day - such a stress and not a healthy or effective way to feel about work - dreading the emails I can't get to. And the tears, arguments, misunderstandings and complaints - all in high supply lately.

It is nice to have my tea made for me daily, and I am grateful for eating with the presenters - a privilege and quite nice.

First time I've actually been cold sleeping, and rainy cold is tough in a tent. I remembered that I have another blanket that I use as a chair pad, and that should help tonight." (January 25)

"A beautiful, sunny day and busy one -

...Amazing to think back just a year ago, when I attended the Ayurveda Conference here - it is again the conference and each night's lecture is about Ayurveda." (January 26)

"Another beautiful, sunny day - meetings and work and the highlight - teaching staff class!

...Next Wednesday, I will teach the intermediate class in the afternoon - excited and a little nervous, but more excited!" (January 27)

"Not slept well past two nights and my supervisor is on a mission to increase numbers and to fix the booking engine - and the constant pushing I feel is starting to wear on me. I missed silent walking meditation today. I'm not sure if I will continue here, and while I think I'd like to write my book here, it is increasingly evident that finding the time while doing karma yoga would be extremely challenging. I have time to consider, but today I also want to keep open other options that would provide me with less stress while I am writing.

I plan to go home for Mom's birthday instead of going to M & M's wedding. It feels like a good decision and will make Mom happy, I'm sure." (January 28)

You might wonder about the mission to increase numbers that I mentioned. The Ashram was created to share yoga and help as many people as possible through yoga, with a broader goal of creating a more peaceful world. In that effort, Swami Vishnudevananda, who founded the Ashram, created a yoga vacation program to provide guests with a place to relax, rejuvenate, and heal from their worldly stresses and problems. He knew that daily yoga classes, healthy fresh vegetarian food, chanting, meditation and educational speakers, plus the healing nature of the pristine ocean would help revitalize those who were open to an Ashram setting and chose to visit. Hundreds of thousands of people have visited the Ashram, and tens of thousands have taken the teacher training to become yoga teachers. Hosting and providing programs for that many people also has a business side to it, as facilities need to be maintained, Bahamian workers need to be paid, karma yogis need to be available, marketing and promotion is needed, and programming provided. Despite that, the priority of the Ashram remains the sharing of the yogic path, as much as possible and with as many people as possible. It was therefore quite natural for Rukmini, as a senior staff member responsible for insuring the continual flow of new guests and yoga teacher trainees, to be concerned about maintaining numbers. My interpretation of her words and her questions were a reflection of my own ego issues of perfectionism. I came to learn this over time and, after some time had passed, I realized that I had often overreacted. My initial reactions, unfortunately, were often negative. Even my supervisor, it seemed, was a 'saint maker' for me.

"Bad night and woke dreaming I was going to the bathroom - had to wash my sheets. I am documenting this recurrence and flash back to my youth and so many nights of sincerely believing I went to the bathroom, when I told it to my mother - the dream was so real. Then I was a little girl, but I can attest to it seeming so real to me now too.

The day itself was busy, full but nothing special that needed recalling. There is much stress around increasing the # of guests at the ashram, and my supervisor keeps pressing with more and more requests of ways to promote and create more buzz and drive the numbers upward. This may be impacting my psyche and causing sleep distress, but the depth of sleep felt good. And while I woke in a panic to get to the bathroom, I also felt as though I got a solid night of sleep.

Very strange why I still have the trouble with my bladder/urinary functioning. I'm hoping that KP will figure it out and the herbs etc. will continue to build my cell structure and improve my health." (January 29)

The bed-wetting incident is not an easy topic to discuss, and definitely not something this "perfectionist" Pitta would have divulged in the past. Believe me, I hesitated to include it in this book. Yet it happened to me for a reason. Why, after so many years of not having such an incident, would it recur? When I was a young girl, my parents had sought answers for this problem, and I was even checked into a hospital for overnight observation and for testing. Nothing was found by the doctors to shed any light. I was simply told to not drink fluids before bed, which was already something I had been doing.

It was a very embarrassing problem to have, and I remember the arguments and tears I shed over not being able to go to sleepovers when I was invited. I insisted that I wouldn't have the problem if I could go to the sleepover, but of course my parents knew that the possibility was high that I would have an accident. Camp experiences as a young child were out of the question too. And while I didn't experience bed-wetting as an adult, I did usually get up every 2-3 hours to go to the bathroom each night. Maybe there were psychological reasons as well, besides the digestive issues at the root of my insomnia? Or maybe my diet and perfectionist temperament impacted the bed-wetting from the time I was a young child? All I can tell you is that the dream was so real that I believed I had gotten up and had gone to the toilet. I was shocked that the small amount of wet that I finally felt had actually happened. I practically ran to the toilet, which was another feat in and of itself, with it finally having turned cool outside. This incident did not make me laugh. It was such a powerful deja-vu to many unpleasant memories.

I'm not sure how this incident will help someone, but I am compelled to include it. It is my loving intention that someone out there will benefit from this rather painful sharing.

ENURESIS - COMMENTARY

By *K P Khalsa*

Having to urinate more often than optimal is a general sign of lack of prana being stored in the body. Mature women often experience this as they begin to produce less estrogen. Temporarily, we use astringent herbs, such as turmeric and bibitaki. Over the long term, this usually improves as ojas (vital force) increases, and the body is more able to keep itself from "leaking" when not appropriate. It is a sign of aggravated "apana", the downward moving energy of the body. In terms of yoga, it can be counteracted by asanas that promote prana and samana, the regulating energy of the midsection of the body.

Padmavati was also taking gokshura, which, over time, tones and supports the urinary tract. It can cause some extra urination at first.

Ayurveda has a very valuable concept that centers on the issue of pre-existing weakness. These areas of potential trouble can be inherited (think familial heart disease) or caused by energy imbalances over the course of life (think tennis elbow). They can, and many times do, overlap. People tend to get injured or develop dosha excess in areas of inherited energy problems. Often today's problem had its roots in these areas of established energy imbalances centered in a specific body part, system or dosha.

As stated above, urinary concerns are quite common in aging women, particularly those who have been pregnant, but there is probably more to this story. Padmavati had unusual difficulties with urinary retention as a child, a classic pre-existing imbalance. While this seemed to dissipate as she matured, it is likely that the underlying imbalance was still there in a less active form. When we began to challenge this issue with some herbs that can stimulate urination, she had some difficulty with urinary urging. This should ultimately resolve as she continues to work on this system. These "hidden" imbalances often take more work to heal than one would think, since the imbalance is less superficially obvious.

SPEEDING UP REALITY

This world is your body. This world is a great school.
This world is your silent teacher.

Swami Sivananda

February and March 2016

Even though I was daily immersed in spiritual practices, did my karma yoga faithfully (and usually to a fault) and had not been killing any of the nature life I tried to co-exist with, I had yet to become a saint! It's a good thing that such an intention was not the goal for this yearlong study. The 'saint makers' were still needed and the "What's Possible?" question continued to be a constant reminder to me of why I was there.

Everything seemed to happen in a 'sped up' fashion, even though life at the Ashram would appear to any observer, including me, to be peaceful and calm. The communal living, the daily churning of our prana through breathing exercises and yoga, the spiritual energy, and the pace of working seven days a week, allowed for our own "stuff" to surface and the lessons to come at us quicker. Dealing with this deeply buried "stuff" meant facing the pain and suffering that accompanies emotional baggage. The beauty of the Yoga and the Ayurveda is that they were working together in my body to force problems to the surface, while simultaneously building new cell composition and new ways of approaching the problems that would replace the old "stuff", whether physical or emotional. Yoga and Ayurveda were both at work on my physical insides, but they also gave me new emotional tools to handle what surfaced. Often the fixing was messy and wasn't immediate, especially for the stronger old habits and buried issues, but I noticed progress nonetheless. Just being able to identify the reaction I had or the thought that came up for no apparent reason was a step in the right direction.

To anyone who knew me in social settings, I was optimistic, energetic, cheerful and generally fun to be around. As a parent, I was loving, fun and nurturing, but I also had another side that was intense, strict, and set very high standards for my children. Anger and frustration often accompanied disappointments from this side of me. And in the work environment, my colleagues had mixed feelings about working with me. I worked very hard at maintaining the optimistic, energetic, cheerful characteristics, and even went further to add passionate, flexible, understanding, open-minded, and a good leader to my work persona. Yet there was still that other side of me that I tried to suppress - the side that set high expectations in a driven manner and liked to control outcomes. I could suppress this part of my nature, but only up to a point. Sometimes I showed up as the flexible, optimistic and understanding leader in the morning, but by mid afternoon, with the annoyances, stresses and disappointments that materialized throughout the day, on an empty stomach and too much coffee, my open-minded and cheerful nature would often have disappeared. When I did manage a few days of maintaining a positive exterior, having suppressed all the annoyances and stress, usually some really minor thing would set me off on a bout of self-pity, anger or resentment, or a combination of all three. A stressed and imbalanced Pitta often ends up overreacting, and not in a pretty and loving way.

My imbalances, as I look back at them today, must have made me appear somewhat of a Jekyll and Hyde character to others. I of course thought of myself as easy to get along with, as loving, kind and generous of spirit, as a good mother, friend and leader. And I genuinely was all of those things, but it wasn't the whole picture. Ayurveda didn't view me as two people or having two sides. There was no Jekyll and Hyde. Instead, Ayurveda recognized me as one person that has certain desirable tendencies and characteristics when balanced, and others that are not so desirable when out of balance.

Ayurveda was teaching me that a balanced Pitta dominant is a sweet-natured, joyous, optimistic, energetic, creative leader who is flexible and open-minded and a pleasure to be around. Ayurveda also taught me that imbalances of Pitta-Vata sparked anger, hostility, self-criticism, irritability, impatience, and resentment and could result in outbursts of temper, argumentative stances (I was certainly known for these!), criticism of others and intolerance. Using Yoga and Ayurveda to achieve balance so that my true nature of love, kindness and generosity would envelop me and be the predominant picture was at the root of my "What's Possible?" quest.

The Ashram presenters continued to astound me with their depth of inquiry and experience. Night after night, I was exposed to enlightening information and intriguing dialogue. And thus far, I had not heard of even one of these presenters before coming to the Ashram. It fascinates me how easy it is to believe that whatever sphere of experience we have is the sphere of experience of everyone. While there is certainly shared and common experience for all humans, the worlds we each experience are vastly different bubbles.

"Last night, John Perkins spoke and was extremely interesting. He was a past economist who advised the US and other country's Presidents and was an Economic Hit Man and Shaman. He's a best selling author of the book Confessions of an Economic Hit Man and Shapeshifting, The World Is As You Dream It.

The day was beautiful temp wise. A nice morning practice and then a full day of meetings and 2 long meetings with Rukmini, one of them walking on the beach with her - so nice." (February 2)

"Beautiful weather and excited to teach today. 4:00 class on the beach platform with about 50 people was a really good class! I used the microphones for the first time and all went really well. I enjoyed teaching and had a few really nice comments after class. I can't wait to teach again :)" (February 3)

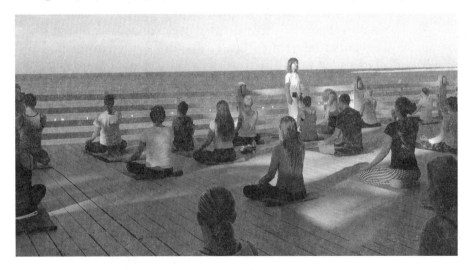

"A busy day of meetings and working on report for Swamiji with Rukmini. Washing my yoga mat was so needed, and I'm glad I finally got around to it..." (February 4)

"Busy day of work - not much disharmony and mostly good and productive day." (February 5)

"Tired in the morning but made it on-time to satsang and had a good yoga practice with Krishnadas teaching - a good start to the day. I did all my laundry today, which was nice and all machines were working and available - so easy to do today. Yoga Nidra (a practice of yogic sleep - a deep relaxation tool for healing, even used for PTSD post traumatic stress disorder in veterans) course starts tomorrow - can't wait to learn this tool for teaching! Tonight's satsang on the 5 Elements and Sound was great. John Beaulieu was hilarious when he told the stories of the 5 Element types of personalities - tonight's satsang was filled with laughter :)" (February 6)

"Today's highlight was mainly getting my blog written and keeping my emails to a minimum with course starting. It was touch and go as to whether I was taking the course or not. Rukmini found out that asana practice was not a part of the training, and she suggested I not take the class. I decided to go ahead and this was the 1st time that I didn't follow her guidance. I could tell she was not happy about my choice. I had already gotten permission, paid for the course and wanted this additional training. There was a special puja, as there is for all courses and the opening session was quite good. Raymond Moody's evening satsang talk about near death experiences was very interesting." (February 7)

"Really cold and damp here again. I slept well but didn't want to get up. I also forgot to take out my contacts, which was pretty amazing that I slept as well as I did. I think the yoga nidra yesterday during the opening session helped. Today's lectures and yoga nidra sessions were good and punctuated by an interesting observation by Andal in my class. When she led me in a yoga nidra session, she suggested my "intention" should be "to unplug", after I told her I planned to do emails in the evening and attend the senior staff meeting during our break for the course. She was right of course, and though I noticed the mounting number of emails when I checked, the sun had come out and made the afternoon yoga nidra session even nicer. The healing from yoga nidra goes deep within, and I think I need this healing too." (February 8)

"...I did not go to the office at all today - trying to remain unplugged. Ruminating some about the iRest yoga nidra teachings of inviting all emotions to tea and learning to 'sit with them', rather than trying to quickly remove or reject them. They also teach that we should welcome everything from horror to sadness to negativity as being a healthy approach - rather than a strictly positive thinking approach and only welcoming in the positive and avoiding the negative. There is some conflict in my mind about yoga's austerities and withdrawal of the senses plus detachment as the main goal of dealing with suffering. Swami H

offered to talk about it, but maybe tomorrow - right now I am preferring some Mauna (silence). I am especially tired and drained - the yoga nidra does not give me energy like asana class does, and it has been 3 days without asana practice. Yet, I feel very relaxed and peaceful.

Two people have commented about evidence of Kapha in me - which is very strange to me. Swami Brahmananda said my composure was Kapha-like, and Ford, one of the iRest leaders, said he saw Kapha in my calmness. Not sure how I feel about this, but calm and composure would be 2 qualities I'd seek to have." (February 9)

"My night was disturbed by my choosing to check emails after satsang. I ended up working for close to an hour and went to bed with thoughts of work...Waking just after 4 am is the worst case scenario for me, as I fall back to sleep and do not want to get up at 5:30 am.

...Today's iRest yoga nidra sessions are interesting, but something in me is feeling the experience as rather draining. Emotions, feelings and deep exploration at least thus far, have not energized or ignited me in any way. It's been nice to see that others have had very good experiences and are not feeling the same draining feeling that I feel.

...The continued cool weather makes the daily bundling up with sweat-shirt and socks and blankets, with the course taught in the open air, call into mind home in some ways - though it's much colder back home and one of the challenges I may have in ever calling Chicago home again. Many karma yogis spend the winter months here at the ashram and in some ways that is appealing. But the peaceful, quiet of the summer here is enticing too - though the high heat and humidity and insects are more challenging. Not sure about anything other than continuing to stay open and trust the right answer will come. I'm still on the "What's Possible?" journey, and I like that path. I'm looking forward to seeing KP Khalsa in person when he's here soon." (February 10)

"Left satsang last night part way through, as I had a feverish night and woke feeling so tired - another cold night. Other than an hour each evening, I've been mostly doing well with unplugging from work. The yoga nidras were so needed today. I slept through most of one and went really deep into relaxation for the other two. Not sure how I'll come out at the end of this." (February 11)

"...I started the morning feeling better, but still not well. It's a little warmer today and sun shone throughout the day :) The yoga nidra that Molly led was great - just a beautiful and cleansing feeling - a good way

to end the course. I worked all afternoon and felt pretty relaxed but not great. By evening satsang I felt better, and I enjoyed it." (February 12)

"Had a much needed, great asana practice in the morning. Sun is shining and I feel wonderful. Today was an overall good day - feeling better. It felt good to feel good." (February 13)

As I write this, it has been many months since I took that iRest yoga nidra course, but I have been led through many yoga nidra sessions since and have also led my own classes of yoga nidra. Mostly, I find that yoga nidra is a refreshing and deeply restful practice. When I took the course, I believe my body was struggling in the cold without appropriate clothing, and that my mind was struggling with that initial disagreement with Rukmini over whether I should take the course. The course sessions took all day, and the amount of material we covered was vast. I used a good amount of energy simply concentrating on learning. Doing the three yoga nidra, deep relaxation sessions every day thrust my mind and body into release mode, allowing them to let go of tensions and concerns. I had plenty of both, mostly work related. Luckily, yoga nidra is so powerful, that by the end, much healing had occurred and I was feeling really good, despite my struggles.

"It doesn't feel at all like Valentine's Day. Another good asana practice and nice day.

For our weekly staff meeting, I led an iRest yoga nidra - they were so thankful and happy to have the added relaxation, as they each are feeling really tired. We've all been working hard.

Time is flying by and I'll need to make some decisions soon - whether to sell my townhouse (at a loss) or continue to rent it, whether to return in May to the ashram after my physical exams in Chicago, for six months? or a year?, whether to seek a publisher for my book or self publish?, whether to do a Go Fund Me to raise money? Lots to think about" (February 14)

"An interesting day - struggled a bit getting going, but a good yoga class had me re-energized. Meetings and work occupied most of the day, but I made time to watch the little video of Aurelia playing in a home made tent and it made me smile. She's so cute! I finally purchased a wedding gift for M & M's wedding and sent the 'No' RSVP note - feel better having that done." (February 15)

"Woke at 4:15 am with horrible diarrhea. Was not able to go to satsang - Rukmini visited me to see if I needed anything and was ok. It was a very slow start to the day. After I showered, I had to do laundry. Luckily machines were available and the process went smoothly. No asana practice today and only ate a little fruit and some rice, plus my

CCF tea and some lemon/ginger tea. I felt weak all day, but I worked and accomplished a fair amount. Exhausted this evening and skipping satsang. I'm going to read Bhagavad Gita now and then go to sleep."
(February 16)

"No satsang this morning - still feel weak and not myself. I worked all day, but no yoga class. I hope to wake tomorrow and feel good. I'm disappointed that more than 10 hours of work today still ended me with 100 emails behind. Tomorrow is KP meeting." (February 17)

"Went to satsang and felt good today. My appetite returned and my energy level was also up. It was a very productive day. I went to Gita chanting tonight for the first time in a couple of weeks - great to see 50 people there, instead of the usual 10.

Some battles of will going on with senior staff - all so serious and yet seems a bit childish and ego filled. How I fit into all this, I'm not sure. I'm just happy to feel good :)" (February 18)

"Day was busy and full of challenges, yet not problematic in terms of handling everything. Interesting struggle I'm having is with team members who are often sick and unlike me, they don't work when they are sick. It frustrates me that these mostly younger people have such different work ethics than mine." (February 19)

Why I continued in this cycle at this point on the journey I don't know. Old habits were apparently really strong. It seems so obvious to me now that maybe if I had stopped working when I was sick, I wouldn't have kept getting sick and I would probably have recovered much quicker. Those whose work ethics I was questioning were not actually sick any more than I was. They simply took the time off to heal that I did not allow myself. Impatience, I realized, was part of my problem here. Just as I had no patience for being sick myself when there was work to be done, I had no patience for others being sick either. I still had lessons to learn from the 'saint makers'.

"Time marches on and the days go by so quickly here. Today was a beautiful weather day and also productive day. Plus I got to teach the afternoon Intermediate Class - a good class on the Garden West platform!

Swami Swaroopananda (the Spiritual Acharya or Leader of the ashram) arrived today, along with Swami Prema and Jnaneshwari - they will join us at the Krishna Das concert tonight. All the senior staff have been busily and happily preparing for the Swamis arrival. Rukmini cooked a special meal for Swamiji's first night back.

Having such good conversations with my office mate lately. I really enjoy working with her." (February 21)

"...Had a good meeting with KP today and he seemed pleased with my progress. Made a hair appointment for trip home for Mom's birthday in March - will be a treat and feel good to feel pretty. Not being attached to my looks is one thing, and a good thing, but generally I still like looking nice. I appreciate beauty. If that's an ego thing, then it's not too clear to me why all the deities are pictured as well dressed and adorned with jewels. Beauty is a positive thing in our world to enjoy and appreciate - just not to the extremes we take it, as is often the case - being consumed with beauty products and procedures is not a good thing either." (February 22)

"Busy day and got lots accomplished ... Team is mostly functioning fine - some computer crashes and personality conflicts, but generally all is ok." (February 23)

"The long walk with Rukmini today was so nice. She wants me to stay and figure out a way to write the book at the ashram. Somehow, I'm not convinced that I could do it while doing karma yoga, and I cannot afford to stay at the ashram as a guest for the months it will take to write the book. And even if I could afford it, I don't think I could just ignore all the work that I would know is there and that needs help doing. I would have to help.

Swamji's Question and Answer session tonight at satsang should be really interesting." (February 25)

"The past 3 nights have been electrical work done during the night and I think the noise from the work has wakened me each night - at least that's what I hope has caused this sudden waking in the middle of the night again. KP also increases some dosages and that might be part of the problem. I'll keep monitoring and let KP know if an issue.

Day went by fast...the workload doesn't seem to ease somehow, even though everyone is busy working and producing well for the most part.

I'm still unsure what I will do at the end of my time in April. The biggest ? is whether I can indeed write the book as I plan to do here.

I submitted a request to the Chicago Perch to see if they'd take on my book project. I'm glad I finally sent off the formal inquiry and trust that whatever is meant to be will be.

I'm now reading the Bhagavad Gita 13X as Rukmini said I should try to do, a chapter a night. Ending so I can now read for 10 minutes." (February 26)

"A very productive day, and things seem under control...." (February 27)

"...The day was productive and I wrote the blog, finished my team update... I am on Chapter 4 of the Gita and feeling good about it." (February 28)

"I had a great yoga class in the morning and then attended the Thai Yoga Massage workshop for part of the time, and I got a nice mini massage in the workshop.

Some ruffled feathers that I didn't expect in a meeting about the pilot and booking engine. Luckily meeting ended up ok, but was not a pleasant start.

Tonight is Sachdev's flute concert which I'm looking forward to - his music is so beautiful and at 82, he can play for 45 minutes straight - just amazing. And he's now making plans to start a music school at the ashram - a man with phenomenal energy.

I leave for home in 9 days - a good break time." (February 29)

"I'm not sure if I'm actually getting better at organizing and am actually catching up, or if it is a fluke.

Two days in a row, I've kept emails down to under 20 and I had 2 good meetings plus taught Yoga today. My TTC buddy arrived today for 3 months of karma yoga - so happy to see her and will be such fun to have her here. She's going to join the Communications Team in April.

Teaching was awesome, and I helped 3 women to learn the headstand after class was over - got them to the 6th step comfortably and they seemed really happy to have the individual teaching. They'll keep practicing until they can easily do the 8th and final step of the headstand.

I'm up to the 11th Discourse (chapter) in the Gita and love taking the time to read each night. It's very relaxing and a nice way to go into meditation at satsang. I teach again tomorrow and Friday :)" (March 1)

I found the spiritual progress of this journey to be the most surprising, as I had no expectations along these lines. Increasingly, the Sadhana became more and more a part of my support system. When I missed a satsang or a yoga class, I noticed it within days. There were definite negative impacts from neglecting these spiritual practices, both on my health and on my psychological wellbeing. The chanting, in particular, was a practice that could notably change my mood and general sense of wellbeing in a very quick and positive way. When I was actively engaged in both satsangs, went to yoga class, ate my meals slowly and in a calm, peaceful fashion, did a little reading from scriptures and took all of the prescribed herbs and supplements, I was physically, mentally and spiritually supported to the fullest.

Usually, on those days, the typical problems that I faced were handled calmly and efficiently. The 'saint makers' brought chuckles and knowing grins to my face, rather than gritted teeth, neck spasms and brow furrowing. The practices were helping me to notice the effects after the fact, and with the lessons of TTC, I understood why the practices were helping. The challenge was still in trying to lessen my ingrained negative reactions, neutralize them, or ideally turn them right around into chuckles and grins. If I could replace the frustrations with joy, the annoyances with smiles, the judgements with love and learn to balance my approach to work - now that would be some amazing progress! At this point in the journey, I knew I still wanted to find out "What's Possible?" in this area too. Realizing that it was indeed a possibility was great progress.

"Generally a good day...one of our key team members may be leaving, and since she does our catalogs and leads the editorial side of things for marketing, it would be a big loss. Time will tell.

My teaching today was really off - not sure why, but I got stuck in the opening prayer and then again in the thanking of the gurus, Swami Sivananda and Swami Vishnudevananda at the end of class. Plus, the microphone was acting up and I struggled with it squeaking when I moved a certain way. It was a nice class overall, but definitely not one of my best efforts. Hopefully, Friday's class will be smoother.

chapter 13 Gita - time to read." (March 2)

"Morning was good...then one of the karma yogis came into the office to complain about two of his office mates - the issues? whether or not food was smelling up the office and whose food was to blame and whether it was ok to have the door opened or door closed - two were too cold with the a/c, so wanted the door open for fresh air, and he wanted to maintain temperature for the video equipment and other equipment in the multi-media office. Four people actually sharing the space makes for frustration and agitation and then venting to me. Two of the off-site professional staff are also struggling to get along and work well together. Both are strong willed women and like to be right.

When I had my Ayurveda massage treatment today, the therapist said she could feel in my body that I wanted to cry. I didn't feel sad, but evidently internally my body senses something is going on.

I've definitely got the added stressor at the moment of taxes and health insurance paperwork and when I will find the time to get both done.

I'm still not sure about staying at the ashram to write the book. I really want it to work, and Rukmini has made some creative proposals about making it work. Yet, I continue to see that the same struggles exist in the ashram that exist elsewhere, and that they are unpredictable. The spiritual anchor of the ashram is an amazing benefit, and I am so grateful for it and for the support I feel on this journey. From one day to the next though, the lessons just keep coming." (March 4)

"Started waking in the night, tired in the morning and finding it tough to get to satsang.

...I taught today and while only 3 people were in class, it was actually quite a good class. One of the students was a new TTC student and I helped her with headstand plus answered questions about Anuloma Viloma after class. They all said they enjoyed the class and liked my energy.

I finished Gita and am starting on the 2nd time." (March 4)

"A day of small frustrations from other people's issues. I'm hopeful that tomorrow's yoga nidra that I will do for the team will help. They need a boost of some kind that brings them back together. Thank goodness for my office mate, as she and I work extremely well together and it is a true blessing. She reminds me of a younger and calmer me." (March 5)

"A day of ups and downs and growing frustration with the continual barrage of additions to my "To Do" list from my supervisor. It's easy enough to just do what I am asked to do. I've been here long enough now to assess more and know that some of the asks are producing chaos and less than optimal working situations for the team. Disrupting the monthly workflow that was discussed and agreed upon, plus staff assigned and appropriate amounts of time allowed for, is ok once in awhile. But the continual insertion of immediate needs when the staff is part-time and already over their contracted hours is not an effective path to be going down. Yet, when the leader of the department say's she wants something done, whether it's in our plans or not, we all try to jump to get it done and please her. The HR issues that then are inevitable when people can't get their regular work done because they are doing the "latest high priority" wears on me and is just emotionally and mentally exhausting." (March 6)

"Feeling tired and knowing Sivaratri is coming - the all night celebration - has me ready to go home for a few days. I'll get some rest. I know

I'll miss the ashram and our diet and yoga classes, but sleeping in a dry and comfortable room even for one hour more each night will be welcome respite...

Good meeting with Royal Caribbean reps and a great teaching experience this afternoon! A couple of the ladies asked when I'd be teaching again :)" (March 7)

"Maha Sivaratri celebration tonight has all karma yogis pitching in to decorate and make Prasad (blessed food) for the night of the celebration of Siva uniting with Shakti - the masculine and feminine aspects of uniting and becoming one with the self and all.

We stayed up all night, chanting pretty much non-stop until 6 am the following morning. We had 5 different pujas (spiritual ceremonies) and the whole platform was elaborately decorated with palms and hand made birds and candles and fruit and other cloth strips hung here and there for color - a pretty spectacular effect when it was done. The Prasad Feast at 6 am had more sweet treats than could possibly be eaten, even though there were 300 of us. 3 lengths of banquet style tables held the many handmade treats. Not much vegan, and everyone was too tired to figure out what was vegan. I really only enjoyed the cinnamon rolls - everything else I tried was too sweet and too rich for me.

I fell asleep during the celebration for a little more than an hour and then I slept after from 6:30 am until 8 am. I had to be ready to leave on the 8:30 am boat to catch the cab and then plane for home." (March 8)

"My day today is all about traveling. At the airport, I managed to work on emails and get them down to about 80 unanswered. I am writing on the plane and plan to stop soon and sleep. I finally got a message and found out that the health insurance issue is resolved. A big relief! Now if I can just get my taxes completed and sent in while I am home, I'll be in fairly good shape. I still need to schedule doctors appointments for the end of the year exams. If I am staying at the ashram to write the book, then I'll need to order more of my herbs and supplements for while I am there. I'm not sure yet if it's meant to be, but so far, no other better option has surfaced." (March 9)

"I was so exhausted that I slept for 7 1/2 hours straight and woke feeling very refreshed! It was so nice to sleep well, and I also had the added plus of a rock star BM this morning hahaha..." (March 10)

My mom's birthday was the reason for the trip, and I was looking forward to celebrating her special day as well as seeing the rest of my family. A surprise visit from my nephew and his girlfriend made the celebration even more fun, and my mom was thrilled to have them with us. The family dinner gathering in honor of my mom was filled with love, laughter and engaging conversation - including, as it was election year, a healthy dose of politics.

My mom worked part-time until she was 84, and she has always been meticulous about caring for her home. She still is an active woman. When she's resting, she's either reading about one of the presidential candidates or past presidents, or she's watching the current political debates. She learned the backgrounds of every candidate, and as a political enthusiast, her favorite companion was Fox News. She usually starts and ends her days watching Fox, and as you may recall from Christmas, my mom's days start before the sun rises. Bill O'Reilly has been one her favorite political commentators, and she's read quite a few of his books.

In the U.S. 2016 presidential election, my mom was supporting Donald Trump. As she put it, she "...normally wouldn't like the harsh rhetoric he's known for", but she believed "...he is a man for these turbulent and troubled times in our world." She most admired his forthright honesty and his strength, and said that she understood his approach of retaliating twice as hard against anyone who attacks him. She believed that in his heart he was a true American who was leading the fight of a righteous war to regain America's greatness.

It was interesting for me to listen and observe during my few days home, especially when my aunt and uncle joined in the debate. I found that I admired the intensity of their support and their dedication to learning whatever they could about the candidates from both parties. Whereas in the past, the political discussions in our house were very painful for me. I rarely shared the opinions of what I deemed to be the extreme conservative views of my family members. I've been a fiscal conservative, but tended to be much more liberal socially than the rest of my family. My former husband and I would cancel out each other's votes and generally laugh about it.

I was completely shut off from TV and the news while at the Ashram in the Bahamas. Occasionally the conversation with the presenters at meal time would bring me up to date on what was going on elsewhere. But, it wasn't a daily dosage of news, as I had been accustomed to before my stay at the Ashram. It was interesting for me to observe how much less attached I was to a strong view about the politics in the U.S. It seemed I was listening to it all with fresh ears and and a fresh mind.

For the first time, it wasn't painful at all. The contrast of worlds I went back and forth between was starkly evident, but it was also becoming evident to me that in both worlds there are many good, loving people who are living life in the best way they know how. I think the balancing effects of the Ayurveda and the purification of my mind from yoga must have been working. I felt less constricted and less entrenched in my own views. This completely new way of viewing the political discussions which have plagued my past adult years was not intentional nor an effort made on my part, in the least. I just heard the conversations and the saw entire situation differently than I ever had before - and it was such a freeing and nice feeling.

"So tired today, with the time change I would have lost an hour anyway, plus Mom panicked and worried that I was going to be late for the time I wanted an Uber pickup (5 am), forgetting we already set the clocks forward and thinking it was 4:30 am when it was only 3:30 am, she knocked on my bedroom door and anxiously called for me to get up, saying I was going to be late! The positive of the early morning was that once again Uber showed up 10 minutes after I searched for a driver, and Willie was great! He shared that he often travels to Puerto Rico, where he owns a home and plans to winter there in the future. His mother lives in the Chicago area, so right now he goes back and forth every month. Another interesting ride with good conversation and on time service too!

I wrote my blog on the plane and finished it up when I got back to the ashram. I had time for a yoga class before dinner. Tonight is a presentation from the Neuroscience Panel - should be interesting. I'm anxious to go to sleep and hope to wake feeling good tomorrow, as it will be a long and busy day. I teach tomorrow afternoon and am looking forward to it!" (March 13)

"I didn't sleep very well, but didn't get up to go to the toilet. Day was all around just ok. I've had a headache all day long - not sure why. Email backlog is huge again and it seems that every email I read is an issue of one kind or another. One of the karma yogis announced that she was leaving earlier than she originally signed up for. She also wants to take a 5 day course before she leaves, which of course will leave her very little time to transition or complete any of her incomplete work. The photographer also wants to take the course too, and she will be leaving, along with another of the staff members sharing the multi-media office. Fewer staff will mean fewer problems, so that may be ok. Until they leave, getting work from them to help the ashram may be a challenge.

I taught today and was a good class, but sun and heat did not help my headache. I'm hoping it isn't stress induced already, as I just got back. If it is stress induced, then the signs of me staying longer at the ashram don't look promising. I'll give it a week, but I'm sure hoping all this drama and work related stress dissipates.

Maybe it was the spraying of OFF in my office tent area last night when swarms of flying bugs showed up when I turned the light on to read the Gita. Flying termites is what I've been told they are, and that they disappear literally overnight." (March 14)

"I woke with still having a headache and had severe pain across my eye and forehead area. My head hurt most of the day. After my Sadhana meeting, my office mate convinced me to go in the ocean - and the 10 or 15 minutes actually did help. The ocean's healing properties are quite powerful at the ashram, and for the life of me, I don't know why I don't go in the ocean more.

The headache wasn't completely gone, but it was less painful. I met with Rukmini today and discussed quite a bit that has needed to be talked about. My headache is a little better this evening, so maybe I'm in the clear now.

I put in a new pair of contacts too, in case I somehow got bug spray on the other contacts. Tomorrow I teach again, which is great!

I am not sure how I'll manage to whittle down the 220 emails to a manageable # but I need to - it's an added pressure.

Deciding on whether to go back home or stay here to write the book is a big decision that for some reason just doesn't seem to be clear to me - " (March 15)

"Teaching went well - enjoy helping others..." (March 16)

"St Patty's Day didn't feel like it at all here - was ok, just different.

I had a Vedic Astrology reading with our Priest today after a rather difficult talk with Rukmini. We ended up fine, but I'm frustrated with staff who go to her and complain, and generally what they are complaining about is basically a directive I am carrying out of hers. She asks me how such and such project is coming along. I then make a direct inquiry of the staff member or karma yogi as to how that project is coming and when it will be complete. I'm then deemed as pushing them and stressing them out. They complain to Rukmini how I'm difficult to work for and that I expect too much. It's circular and not a healthy pattern for staff to get into. Similar to kids in a household running to complain about the other parent. If those parents don't stick together and have a united front, the cycle never ends. It felt like that to me at the moment of our discussion. Fortunately, we agreed that we needed to stay united in our approach to the leadership.

My meeting with the Priest was quite interesting - a whole hour and lots of specific suggestions. I took notes and recorded it, as I'll need to re-listen to it. He did not see me writing the book at the ashram. I'd definitely be back at the ashram and he even said I'd be a presenter in the future, but he saw me leaving in May for at least a few months."
(March 17)

"...woke feeling pretty good - self yoga practice, breakfast and full day of work and then teaching. Mishap with teaching, as I lost track of time and forgot my watch - had to run back to my tent to get the watch and then didn't have time to get cushions for people to use while sitting yogi style to elevate their hips. I started the class with Savasana and had people nicely relaxed, even adjusting shoulders and giving a nice start for the class. When we sat up to do the prayers that is when I realized I hadn't gotten the cushions, and so I went next door to get some for everyone. One of the more regular, multi-year karma yogis gave me an annoyed look and left to join another class. She didn't like the disruption of the flow of the start of class, I'm assuming. Oh well. The rest of the class went well and people seemed happy with it.

I've got a new idea to increase #s concerning karma yogis that I want to share with Rukmini - we'll see how it flies." (March 18)

"My mind has been too focused on work related "must do" pressures and - not feeling positive about it -

Though today's productivity lessened the stress dramatically, as I finally completed and sent out taxes, paid my last 2 premiums to Blue Cross, Blue Shield (I mistakenly missed a payment) and set up automatic payments now that I know the correct payment amount, finished my blog and finally sent a text to family about Gopi Kallayil's book, which I've been meaning to do :)" (March 20)

One of the more challenging elements about living at the Ashram for a year was trying to keep up with personal needs. The senior, full time staff who live permanently at the Ashram have all of their needs taken care of within the Ashram environment. Visits home and other non-Ashram related activities were few and far between for them. Most of the other karma yogis were 'checked out' of their home life for 1-3 months, which was not easy by any means, but easier. The few I met who came for stints of 6 months had been doing so for a number of years, and had developed routines and back-up support. So, my situation of a year was a bit unusual. Of course, if I didn't have the imbalanced, workaholic tendencies so deeply inbred in me, I would have attended to what I needed to, when I needed to do it. There were no time clocks to punch and no evaluations I had to worry about being subjected to, nor was there any chance that I was going to get fired. Yet I was driven much the same as if all those pressures existed. I was my own worst enemy and a very strong opponent to deal with.

"...For the negativity in me to be growing daily is not a good sign." (March 21)

"...I mentioned to Swami Brahmananda that I may not be here in June when he said I could take his Meditation Course (which I wanted to take). He seemed surprised and said "Where else would you be?" I said that I want to write my book, and Rukmini piped in with you can do it - I said quietly that I didn't really think so.

I'm glad to have at least started conversations about leaving with them. KP will be here tomorrow and I'm looking forward to seeing him." (March 22)

"I taught yoga this morning and it was a great class - such a nice group and so many said the class was helpful and thanked me - felt good.

I attended KP's workshop and met his wife. She seems really nice. It was good to see him! Tonight is KP's satsang talk - should be good." (March 23)

"Taught yoga today, and Krishnadas took my class and then provided lots of feedback. Overall impression was of a good class and good flow of energy in the class...Mostly comments were positive and was great to know what could have been better and get his suggestions. They will help me improve next time.

I also met with KP about the book, and he confirmed his commitment to collaborate on the project. So excited that he will also reach out to 2 publishers he knows to see if they'd be interested in publishing the book! Our talk was nice and a big help - good to catch up in person and gave me a chance to thank him in person too. His wife, Jagadeesh also sat in on part of the meeting. I think she found the story of the past year to be interesting, and she will be supportive of KP continuing to help me.

KP seemed to think rainy season in Thailand to write the book might be a perfect place, when I shared rather jokingly about Kam Thye Chow suggesting that I should go to Thailand for inspiration and a good place to write, and that other mentions of Thailand had recently surfaced, and the Vedic reading of the Priest said I would visit Thailand.

It's been a long day - Rukmini's birthday and lots of celebrating, plus a great kirtan concert tonight - but I'm tired." (March 25)

"Was warm sleeping last night and not a good night's rest. I took Krishnadas' yoga class, and it felt really good. I enjoyed breakfast and had time to chat more with KP and Jagdish - such nice people.

Day was ok - one of the karma yogis chose today to let me know how mean she felt I had been to her. It was a long and tough hour of letting her vent and some back and forth of sharing viewpoints. The end result was peace, but I was exhausted by it and emotionally drained, and I'm guessing she was too. It was a sad situation from my perspective of my trying to be so sympathetic and supportive with struggles she had in the early months of her arrival, then eventually frustration and disharmony were the overriding feelings for both of us in the last month.

My expectations for this karma yogi, Rukmini's expressed requests for her work output and the actual output were not close to the same. She was miserable and so was I. My assessment was that she would benefit by learning to focus and create more product. Her assessment was that she didn't have enough guidance and at times had conflicting guidance on her projects. I on the other hand, needed to revise my expectations, not take things personally and should expect that overseeing karma yogis would continue to be challenging. "Saint making" work for sure in this case.

Kirtan concert was too loud and funky chanting for me - lots of others enjoyed it. Tired!" (March 26)

"Beautiful Easter sunrise service with the Gospel Choir from Trinity Baptist Church and the Bishop presiding. An interesting and unique service followed by a HUGE Easter Feast that was really incredible to see and eat.

Royal Caribbean Majesty of the Seas Day Excursion Director and one of her staff were on property today for inspection. We fed them, gave them a tour and answered questions. They took lots of photos and were positive about their experience. They will file a report and then likely 1 more visit will yet be necessary before the partnership will be finalized - a long, slow process.

I worked well with the karma yogi who called me mean yesterday, as she interviewed me for a video on Essentials Courses. No yoga today - not good - but a pretty nice day." (March 27)

"...catching up on work and trying to decide on where to write my book. I can't picture writing it somewhere other than here, and yet the signals are clear that trying to do karma yoga and write will be conflicting...I'm tired of putting in extra hours and plan to cut back in the next few weeks to see if I can regain my positive spirit being here with the work I do. Otherwise, I'm going to take a break from here and regroup for the book writing phase of my journey." (March 28)

"Waking during the night is not tolerable to me anymore, and I'm doing it again...I booked my flights for Arkansas and Chicago - travel

to John's on May 7 and to Chicago on May 14, my brother's birthday. Will be good to go home." (March 29)

"Pretty regular day - ...each day, I feel less inclined to return, as Rukmini asked me to do, from June - December. Helping out and delaying the writing of my book was the request at our most recent meeting. I'm not sure Thailand is it, but that thought excites me and seems pretty interesting, and it would definitely be nice to only focus on my writing for a few months. I do not want to delay the writing of the book.

I had to cancel my flights, as I booked them to the wrong airport - yikes! At least I caught it in time and cancelled with no penalty.." (March 30)

"Felt better this morning - taught morning yoga class. 60 or so people on the beach platform - a full class. Was fun and I helped another woman after class with headstand. Rebooked flights and will fly to John's on May 6 and home to Chicago on May 14. Feeling tired this evening - TTC graduation tonight." (March 31)

As I relived these journal entries, I realized that the struggle I was having about where to write the book - and more specifically, the struggle of whether to write the book at the Ashram - reminded me of another time, when I was readying myself to leave home for the first time and go off to college. It was a time of separation that was prefaced with months of arguments, frustration and misery with my siblings and parents. In order for me to be able to separate from the home and people I loved, I created an atmosphere of disharmony. It's easier to leave someplace that you want to leave than to leave a place of comfort, love and happiness.

This tug of war that I was feeling at the Ashram was similar. I think I realized pretty early on that doing karma yoga plus trying to write was not going to be a good plan. I needed a singular focus, and I didn't trust my own tendencies to volunteer to help when help was needed. But I was also really torn about not having the environment of the Ashram and spiritual support while I was writing the book. By now, I understood the substantial benefits that I'd gained by being at the Ashram, and I knew that the support was very powerful. I also really enjoyed being part of the long-term staff and cared dearly for each of them. I genuinely liked being at the Ashram. Yet envisioning a workable plan for writing the book there wasn't coming to me. So I began to create that same atmosphere of disharmony, in order to make the decision to leave easier. Rukmini, who I truly love, respect and admire, was all of a sudden a demanding supervisor in my mind. I focused on the feelings of tiredness, or the personnel issues, or my old favorite, the email counts.

A new approach I'd learned from yoga - when things don't flow easily, wait and trust that another path will present itself.

NEARING THE FINISH LINE

Put your heart, mind, and soul into even your smallest acts.
This is the secret of success.

Swami Sivananda

April 2016

You might think, after reading the last few months of my journal entries, that I was anxious to leave the Ashram. I really was not. I had daily challenges and those challenges tended to make it into my journal entries, but my general feeling about the Ashram was one of gratitude for all that I was experiencing and learning. My personal growth was very significant in all areas, from physical to emotional and mental, to spiritual.

As it turned out, apart from the TTC month of November, April was my most significant month of the year. It was by far the most difficult, but also the most rewarding.

It started off with a fascinating series of satsangs with John Douillard, who spoke about nutrition and Ayurveda. He enlightened us about a 60-year old mistake by the US Health Department, which involved advocating the removal of fat and cholesterol from the diet of Americans, including schoolchildren, and substituting processed fats and sugars instead. The Low Fat and Fat Free craze that has dominated the American diet ever since was actually based on a flawed study. It resulted in the trend toward obesity that is now worse than ever and set us up for the tremendous increase in diabetes prevalent today.

He also spoke of the concerns he had about the similar craze of eating gluten-free, as most gluten-free products are highly processed. Humans have eaten wheat for the past 3.4 million years, and our genetics are predisposed to process wheats. In contrast, humans have eaten meat for only 500,000 years, and originally only out of necessity when lands were not producing the food that man needed to survive. Douillard further added that to be able to eat wheat means you have a good digestive system. Digestion and detoxification are closely related, and elimination of too many foods can cause problems with natural detoxification in the body. He suggested that many of those who are eating gluten-free diets today should instead be looking at what's wrong with their digestive system, in order to get to the root cause of their problems with certain foods.

Of course, I found the talks interesting and a great start to April.

"Past 3 days have had on and off diarrhea and is beyond frustrating. Have washed 3 pair of pants, one or two each day from accidents and on one day, I soaked 2 pair of pants in bleach without water for many hours (was rushing and forgot to come back and add the water). I didn't have time to wash and left the pants overnight - they were shredded, with huge holes and unusable by morning. I had to buy new pants, so I'd have pants to teach in. We have to wear all white pants and our yellow shirts when we teach. By the third day, Rukmini gave me a couple pills that kind of look like Pepto Bismal. KP thinks I caught a bug of some kind. It was also in the 90's past few days too, so heat hasn't helped.

Tonight is another talk by John Douillard - he's pretty fun to listen to, so I'll enjoy." (April 3)

"No diarrhea for past few days, but nearly 50 people in 2 days had intestinal problems - mostly vomiting and flu symptoms. Glad I didn't have that! They have been quarantined since yesterday, as a precaution, with the Zika virus outbreaks a problem in the U.S. and the UK. The ashram is doing all it can to prevent spread of the flu to the guests and to take care of the karma yogis. I've been impressed with their approach.

I'm exhausted from covering the Ashram Tour, opening and closing workshops with prayers and helping presenters in their workshops, making daily announcements, teaching 2 classes each day and doing the evening tour. It might have been ok if I had managed to have more than 15 minutes of asana practice today. Yesterday, I had 30 minutes, and today I planned on an hour. Then I had a last minute request from

Rukmini to make folders, with pictures glued to the front, for 33 students for her Bhagavad Gita class. I had planned to start asanas in about 10 minutes from her request. Needless to say, I grumbled as I made her folders. Lately, Rukmini is driving herself and me/her team, and I was reminded of myself and how I no longer wanted to be." (April 7)

"Today was generally a good day. The intermediate class on the beach went well, as did the 3 sets of breakfast time announcements and the tour - all were going well - then I opened the workshop and stayed to assist for the Tibetan Lama's talk on meditation - quite interesting - and then I did the closing prayers.

Sometime during the morning, Rukmini decided to add bell ringing to my duty list and when she made the request to me, as she herself was rushing to teach a class, my already elevated Pitta, from heat and running from activity to activity to cover for others who were sick, struggled to not explode. I complained in front of Krishnadas, which wasn't the best, but I couldn't take one more Rukmini add-on and said so.

After an hour of personal yoga on the Vishnu Platform by the water, I felt much better and really enjoyed the afternoon yoga class that I taught - a really nice group and great energy.

I teach in the morning again and then I think I'll get a break." (April 8)

"About 40 people are still in quarantine - so the extra duties continue. I'm losing steam but still really enjoying teaching and tours in particular. I've just ignored Rukmini's questions about any deadlines we may be missing while I cannot work at all in the office. Today I just said that whatever is waiting in the office for me, has to wait. I have no more capacity than what I am giving.

I took Narayani's afternoon yoga class after no classes for 10 days and it was like a heaven sent practice for me :)" (April 9)

"I taught this morning and did my own shortened yoga practice on the dock - did not have to do tours or announcements.

I led my first workshop today - an asana workshop - only 4 people who came, but it was a good workshop and I felt each of the attendees were happy with the progress they made during the session. I taught Intermediate class on Bay Platform in the afternoon.

A guest who has been coming to the ashram for 10 years commented after class that he really liked how I taught. He had taken a few of my classes during his week visit and liked my instructions. He appreciated my counting and my letting them know the # of repetitions we would do - all things I learned from taking Krishnadas' classes, that I personally liked. Some instructors give fewer instructions, especially in the intermediate classes. Not considering myself a seasoned practitioner, I was happy to hear that he, who was a longtime Sivananda practitioner still liked the guidance of the instruction. Was nice affirmation that my teaching was helpful." (April 10)

"I didn't go to satsang - slept until 7:30 and then quickly showered and went to the Beginner's class. Class was good, gentle and I needed a break.

Worked in the office all day and did some laundry too - felt good to start catching up.

Adam informed me that The Chicago Perch was not a likely option for my book - a bit disappointing, but must not be the way I'm meant to publish the book.

Madhavi Molly speaks tonight and Richard Miller - originator of iRest yoga nidra is also here. I hope to take a yoga nidra session with him." (April 11)

During the time of the quarantine, the karma yogis with symptoms were not allowed to mingle with others on the property. Food, water and anything else they needed were brought to them in their tents until they fully recovered and showed no symptoms for a full three days.

It meant that those of us who were not sick were covering in all sorts of ways. For me, it meant that I spent no time in the office. As already mentioned in a journal entry, I had a packed schedule and was covering for a few different people. Everyone else at the Ashram had similarly packed schedules and added duties. It was an exhausting week, and yet so much of it was fun.

It was an opportunity to teach beginner's classes, intermediate classes, and even the asana workshop, which was a first for me. On a typical schedule, I only taught 2-3 times in a week. Now, with teaching twice a day, each class was an affirmation of how much I loved to teach. Guests were generous with their kind words and acknowledgement of my classes being good experiences for them. I also got to know the guests in my classes, as I saw them every day. I was happy that the teaching was positive for them, and that I was able in a small way to be part of their practice.

The tours were also fun. Being able to share about the Ashram with newly arriving guests was a labor of love, while opening and closing workshops and making the announcements were a nice change of pace for me. Everything, except the Gita folders and bell ringing, was done with a really positive and good heart, and what I remember most about this crazy time period was that I felt incredibly joyful, so much of the time! I could feel myself smiling more, and my heart felt light. Others noticed it too and commented about my looking radiant.

Yes, I grumbled about the Gita folders. And yes, I lost it when the bell ringing request sounded to my imbalanced Pitta ears like a demand, instead of the true call for help that it really was. The funny thing, as I look back at it, was that the bell ringing was so much easier than I imagined it to be. And I could have said 'no'. It just didn't occur to me.

Overall though, my mood was great, and I was happy. Somehow this stress felt different. I wish I could report that my body reacted as positively as my mind and spirit did. It took awhile to notice the effects, but eventually they showed up.

> *"...I did my own yoga practice on the dock - was very nice. The day was busy, and I felt honored to open the workshop for Richard Miller. I also got to stay and hear him speak - such a calm, peaceful and wise man.*

> *After the workshop, I chatted with my friend and colleague, Madhavi Molly a bit and shared that I still hadn't decided for certain where I was going to write my book. We both knew the demands and unpredictability of karma yoga, and she also thought writing the book while at the ashram would be really tough. I told her about Kam Thye Chow suggesting I go to Thailand to write my book, and that I recently had been having these random people mention Thailand in conversation. The most interesting one was the woman who took my yoga class and then came up afterwards to thank me and share that she was going to be in the next TTC class. We continued our conversation, and I found out that she too had worked in government. Her federal government job had taken her to Afghanistan at one point and then she continued to talk about her rest and relaxation week that was provided after such a deployment, and that she chose to do hers... in Thailand. She liked Thailand so much that she returned there to do a Yoga Training there. Now she decided she wanted to get a more classical training and was taking the Sivananda Teacher Training.*

> *Madhavi agreed that Thailand was trying to get on my radar screen. I asked Madhavi if she had any contacts there. She didn't, but then she called over Richard Miller, and wouldn't you know it - he and his son had just returned from a two week trip to....Thailand :) I asked him about Chiang Mai, and he had been there and also suggested a place called Tak, with a 200 person yoga community that he visited. He sent an email and made a connection to his friends that had led the group trip he and his son had been on. His friend, Michael started the yoga group. I'm excited to see where this leads.*

KP met with his publisher, Lotus Press today." (April 12)

"Yoga class with Madhavi was so great - relaxing and yet energizing - Sivananda style with quite a bit of variation and modifications.

I worked most of the day, but also fit in writing an email introduction to Lotus Press as KP suggested I do. The draft is rough but I sent it off, as it has been a couple days since KP made the request. Will need to polish it, if I am going in the right direction.

I heard from Richard's Thailand friend, Michael.

Sat Bir Singh Khalsa is back at the ashram and talking about the science side of meditation and yoga practice. He's the assistant professor and researcher from Harvard - was an interesting talk." (April 13)

"What a fabulous day! Weather is perfect - yoga again with Madhavi was beautiful and even more healing than the day before. Hoping that SriDevi Jennie will find the couple of herbs that I need while she's home. I want to make sure that I take what I need for the last 2 weeks.

I had an Ayurveda massage treatment today with Iswari, who is an expert and teacher of Marma Points (pressure points). She studied with and now teaches in India with Dr. Vasant Lad, James Tennant's (of Tejas Yoga in Chicago) guru - what a small world in the vastness of life.

I also learned that the publisher KP is talking to, Lotus Press, was founded by a disciple of Sri Aurobindo, whose methodology was the guide for the book Fire of Love that Paul read to us during Restorative Yoga.

This afternoon, after a shower, I will be in Richard Miller's iRest yoga nidra session - then a puja, dinner and Madhavi speaking tonight. Wow - a beautiful day!" (April 14)

You may recall that I had received a spiritual name in early July. Everyone at the Ashram called me Padmavati. 'Padma' means 'lotus' in Sanskrit, and the name itself means 'possessing Lotuses'. So, from the start, I was intrigued by the name of one of the publishing companies KP suggested for our book. When I learned that Lotus Press was founded by a disciple of Sri Aurobindo, I was more than intrigued.

My Restorative Yoga teacher from Tejas Yoga Studio back home in Chicago, Paul Hnatiw, used to read to us from his guru's book, Fire of Love, while we held poses for 10 minutes. This is one of the few yoga books I owned before coming to the Ashram. I loved the stories Paul shared from this book by Aadil Palkhivala, which was devoted to Sri Aurobindo's methodology. At the time, I knew few of the renowned yogis except Sri Aurobindo, and I had spent many blissful moments listening to his messages. Now I stayed open and trusted that what was meant to happen would, but inside me I felt a spark.

Following Richard's endorsement of Thailand and after the email connection was made with Richard's friend, Michael, about Chiang Mai, I pretty much decided that I was meant to go to Thailand. It was calling to me. I was certainly getting enough signals pointing me in that direction. During the yoga nidra that Richard Miller led, I meditated on it, and I knew my answer to when and where I would write this book.

"I begin teaching Essentials 1 today. Just found out yesterday afternoon. I will love doing this! I have 6 students in the course - a very nice group. We had an opening puja ceremony at the Vana Duga Temple (temple in the woods), plus a 2 hour yoga class and 1 1/2 hour lecture.

Prepping and then teaching took most of my day today. I did my own yoga for an hour and heard from MH, my tax preparer that he doesn't have all the forms he needs to submit my taxes. Today is the deadline.

I spent time searching the insurance and government websites and had no success locating the forms, and Mom didn't have anything mailed to her house. Will have to get an extension for my taxes - ugh.

I'm tired but invigorated by the teaching - a nice satsang tonight of music by Shimsai." (April 15)

"Teaching again...After senior staff meeting, I talked with Rukmini and told her I'd decided I was definitely leaving and not delaying the writing of the book. It felt like a huge weighted had been lifted, when I shared with her that I would be going to Thailand and would start writing the book the beginning of June. She was disappointed but took the news well.

No yoga today has me rather sore, but still loving teaching :)" (April 16)

"Full day - teaching Essentials, then graduation puja, then writing of my blog and then teaching intermediate class on the Bay Platform - a full class with Teresa, our new project coordinator taking the class - met her after class for the first time in person. Was a great class and nice comments afterward - helped a guy with his Scorpion and a woman with headstand. Love this!

Science and NonDuality Conference had interesting presentation on consciousness at tonight's satsang." (April 17)

"Spent lots of time with Teresa today and tried to get taxes straightened out - no luck, even with Mom, John and even Mike (my former spouse) trying to help out - was really nice of them to do.

I did yoga twice, as Rukmini Ali, my TTC friend, was teaching a staff class and I wanted to support her. My body is feeling rather achey - not sure why? Looking forward to satsang talk tonight and a good night's sleep." (April 18)

"Generally was a good day - meetings with contracted staff much of the day, with everyone on-site and off-site meeting each other in person. I took staff class with Jagadeshwari today and she asked me to stay after to talk with her. It was a nice conversation and she was grateful for feedback on her teaching - I was happy to give it. She will be a great teacher.

My right buttock and back of leg are sore for some reason - not sure of the 'why?' but am hoping I'll feel back to normal soon. Sri Devi Jennie helped make some herb powder capsules for me - so sweet of her to do. She's looking healthy and happy after her visit home.

...I'm substitute teaching in the morning intermediate class - wish it were afternoon, but I'm happy to have another opportunity to teach." (April 19)

"I woke feeling pretty good today and really enjoyed morning satsang with Nirmala and Satyadev. Teaching on the Bay to a packed platform was a nice boost to the day, and one of the guests shared with me that she liked my class very much - always nice to hear.

The rest of the day was filled with meetings and office work, but a very good day.

Afternoon personal yoga on Vishnu platform was nice and needed. I'm still experiencing pain in my right buttock and down right leg - so strange to feel this pain when I've been pain free for so long.

Not set on Thailand plans, but hope to get them solidified soon. Each day flies by and knowing this year and study has nearly ended feels so strange to me - it's been quite the journey - " (April 20)

"Passover - a full day with Yoga Teacher Reunion classes, meetings and catching up with karma yoga work. My butt cheek, lower back and sciatic nerve are still bothering me - a nagging in the background kind of pain - interesting why we push ourselves so often to the point of pain before easing up.

So grateful for Narayani giving me a Thai Yoga style massage to help with my hip pain.

Everyone helped out with the preparations for Passover, and I helped with cleaning tables, ironing table cloths, carrying out large trays of food and serving food during the evening feast.

It was an amazing experience that went to midnight - 250 people, dressed in our best yogi clothes, with 15 different songs to sing as part of the ceremonies and enough readings for most of us to participate with reading 2 passages each. The Feast was huge and lots of delicious kosher foods were served. Everyone had fun -

There were 2 symbolic ceremonies that started the night before - a candle lit search for leaven bread and then the next morning, a burning/fire ritual to burn the leaven bread pieces, symbolizing the ego - removing the ego to allow for the new Non Slave persona to arise. The 400 years of Jewish slavery and bondage culminated on the night of Passover, when Ramses, Pharaoh of Egypt told the Israelites to leave, after Moses' continual request of the Pharaoh to 'let my people go' and the ensuing plagues that eventually took the lives of the 1st born Egyptian males and Ramses' son died.

The whole night I kept remembering the movies 10 Commandments and Ben Hur. I had seen these movies many times, but until that night at the ashram, I hadn't really put 2 + 2 together, as I had always watched the films in a Christian frame of mind - was interesting to notice how oblivious I had been to other cultures and faiths." (April 22)

"Tired and still sore, but doing everything - enjoyed a gentle yoga practice on Vishnu platform...Staff meeting had me realizing just how soon I will be leaving - really seems strange...I'm working on transition documents for Rukmini, trying to stay calm, as Rukmini is preparing to leave for the EBM (Sivananda International Board Meeting) - readying for the hand off. I'm ready for a new adventure, and yet, I know I will return here at some point." (April 23)

"...no time to investigate the information that Michael sent about Thailand - hoping to have a little time after Rukmini leaves." (April 24)

"hip sore..." (April 25)

"Beautiful, meditative yoga class with Surya this morning - really relaxing and seemed to help hip a bit.

Very busy day, helping Rukmini with her last class - copies, hole punching, printing the EBM report and finalizing all the info for the transition plus gathering International Day of Yoga materials for the June event to hand off to Sri Devi." (April 26)

As I reread all of the entries for this month, it was so obvious that I had put strain on my body when I covered for the 10 or so days during the flu outbreak. What I really believe was the underlying reason for the hip and sciatic problem, though, was the tension that had led up to April with not knowing whether I was staying at the Ashram or not. It was an emotionally draining time, and I felt a heavy weight of burden in believing that I'd disappoint Rukmini who tried so hard to help me stay. This mental stress, coupled with a weakened body, resulted in the physical misery I was feeling as I was approaching the end of the study.

An interesting statistic that presenter Joe Dispenza shared with us: typically, we have 60,000-70,000 thoughts per day..........and 90% of them are the same as the day before. I hadn't ever thought about the number of thoughts that were identical from one day to the next, but in reality, from the moment we wake until we go to sleep, the thoughts are rote and the same. When they are worrisome thoughts or negative thoughts, the groove formed in our mind can result in quite a bit of suffering. We create life habits based on this daily repetition of the same thoughts, and then the same ensuing actions that follow. I'd learned about detachment from thoughts and made progress in this area, but I still had feelings of attachment to Rukmini, to the Ashram, and to others at the Ashram. After only a year of learning these lessons, it was perhaps inevitable.

My mental and spiritual states were quite good. The buoyant feelings of love from teaching yoga each day were providing me with good energy, so I could keep working and keep helping Rukmini until she left. And the daily Sadhana that I was adhering to was fueling that love, so I could keep giving to the yoga students. As my departure neared, I had an overriding feeling of inner peace and calm on most days. I had come a long way from where I started.

"Saw Rukmini off at 7:25 am - she and Swami Swaroopananda left for the EBM meeting in Canada. I had tears as she left. I would be gone before she returned from Canada. I gave her and Swamiji nice cards and hugged Rukmini. My love and admiration of her welled up inside me.

Swami Prema was not going to the meeting. She invited me to have a conversation with her, but unfortunately, I did not have time then. Perhaps I should have made the time and delayed my meeting. Another time.

I got an appointment due to a rare cancellation for an Ayurveda Shirodhara massage treatment with Iswari - what a treat and perfect to help with my hip. I can't believe Rukmini is gone." (April 27)

"...not a very restful night...I assisted teaching yoga again today with the juice fast group. It was a challenge working with the senior teacher, but eventually we worked out a system... Teaching in the mornings really throws off my physical body, without starting with yoga for myself, but I love the teaching - " (April 28)

"Teaching the juice fast group for 8 days is great! Such a nice group, and I am enjoying helping them through this fast with gentle yoga each morning.

I gave the basket from my Mother's Day flowers to Parvati, and told her I pictured her with flowers in the basket - she said she would fill the basket with flowers and bring it to the dock to greet me when I return to the ashram :) It was a nice last staff meeting and good farewell.

I'm doing the evening and morning satsang announcements as part of my duties, since Rukmini and Minakshi are gone to Canada for the EBM meeting.

I wrote my last blog of the study - so hard to believe it has been a year already." (May 1)

"Announcements, teaching and lots of work done today - am catching up - and have hair appointment scheduled.

Teaching the detox group has been very nice. Today, I did a yoga nidra practice with them, and they really enjoyed it.

...I'm increasingly looking forward to some air conditioning and a less regimented schedule. The trip to Thailand will be wonderful and give me some time to regroup a bit. Tired but struggling with heat the past couple of nights." (May 2)

"The days go by in a flash, I'm so busy - but I am taking time to pause and note and appreciate so much and so many here at the ashram.

Announcements, opening and closing workshops, plus satsang presenting the speakers and sharing the daily schedule have all been fun. I make mistakes, but Swami Prema and others have told me that they like my energy - so it's a nice way to be leaving some of my energy at the ashram. I've gotten so much energy from the daily sadhana here, and I will really miss it and miss so many people.

My juice fast group is doing so well - each of them are progressing in their practice and gaining strength, flexibility and confidence. So fun to observe.

I filled in for Sri Devi doing the tour and announcements and I felt I barely had a moment of slow down - but it was a good day!" (May 3)

"Nice teaching experience with juice fast group -

A quick breakfast and then went to the dock to say goodbye to Sri Devi Jennie - such a beautiful spirit. Nirmala left today too, and it was nice to see how much she calmed down from when she arrived. She's a bundle of energy and also a bright light, searching for her worldly happiness. I may see her in Chicago.

Getting excited to go to John's and Beatrice's home and spend time with little Vivi. I hope the transition home will be a good one.

Flights are booked - I leave for Thailand on May 25th and arrive in Chiang Mai on May 27th, with a stopover in Abu Dhabi.

I know that I'm not interested in returning to the fast paced lifestyle that once felt so right to me.

The calm and peace and balance of yoga are much more aligned with how I want to lead my life. I want to teach and continue to purify my heart and mind and radiate love and peace to all I encounter." (May 4)

One of my favorite presenters during the year - and one that embodied many of the lessons I learned - was Gopi Kallayil, the Chief Evangelist Brand Marketing for Google. He shared some fascinating statistics and noted that there were 7.2 billion mobile devices as of February 2015, a greater number for the first time in history than the 7.1 billion people on planet Earth. He jokingly referred to cell phones as "weapons of mass distraction" and he shared his story about bringing yoga to Google. Gopi is also a Sivananda Yoga Teacher, trained at the Dhanwantari Ashram in India. He brought yoga to Google by offering to lead a class each week for free to any Google employees interested in joining him. It has been more than 10 years, and that class continues still; today, there are 38,000 Google employees daily taking yoga classes being offered at their workplaces. Not long ago, at a large employee conference, 11,600 Google staff were in 1 room doing standing asanas. It was the largest indoor gathering of yoga in the U.S. and the third largest in the world. Gopi has definitely influenced and taught many. After completing his TTC, he committed himself to sharing yoga with as many people as possible, just as Swami Vishnudevananda, the founder of the Sivananda Teacher Training Course and Gopi's TTC teacher, sought to do. The overall mission was to bring more peace to the world through fostering peace within each individual.

Part of what I've learned over this year, and what Gopi embodied, is an approach of example and outreach - living the teachings and inviting others to join in, rather than simply identifying someone else as needing better health or less stress or more sleep and offering to "fix them". Only if we ourselves choose to bring more peace, more health, more sleep, and more love into our lives, is it possible to bring about change. Wider change must start from within ourselves. That is why Swami Vishnu said the only real way to peace is through individual peace. It cannot be forced upon others, whether individuals or countries. He taught us that when we ourselves are peaceful, loving and healthy, we will radiate those qualities outward and our energy will have a positive impact on all around us. I believe this is true.

"My last day teaching the juice fast group - was a good class - graduation was really nice too, and the students were very sweet and so appreciative. Even Richard stopped me and expressed his gratitude for the yoga class.

I had a full day continuing to cover for people and starting to pack. It was more difficult than I anticipated, as I had accumulated more books and teaching binders and manuals that were bulky and heavy.

Swami Brahmananda stopped me before dinner and asked me to come to the Vishnu platform at 7 pm after dinner, which I did.

Sri Devi and Rukmini had organized a surprise farewell for me with a beautifully decorated vegan cake that Rhada, a karma yogi friend made. Sri Devi had found the recipe online. It was quite a sweet treat and I could taste the love that was put into it. Senior staff and others were there. Savitri Devi handmade beautiful cards that were signed by many, and I received a gift - the Upanishads Letters Book (more weight for my suitcase LOL), a beautiful book of Swami Sivananda's letters that Swami Vishnu compiled - a perfect gift that I will love having. After prayers and blessings and a few heartfelt expressed sentiments, we all enjoyed the cake.

Rukmini called from Canada during the celebration. I called her back when I went to the office right after the gathering and talked to her for awhile and thanked her for all she'd done for me throughout the year. I told her and all at the party, that I love them and I do.

The last evening satsang was a panel on Spirituality, as part of the Heart and Mind Symposium. Dr. Daniel Drubach, a neurosurgeon at Mayo Clinic, and Iswara closed the evening with beautiful guitar and violin music. A perfect last satsang.

I hugged Swami Prema, who is so amazing and full of love, and then I went to my tent to finish packing. It took me until quite late to get my packing in order.

In the morning I finished up and did some cleaning to leave the tent ready for the next person. I dropped off my sheets in the bins, took out the trash and gave keys to Saraswati. Surya, a woman who radiates sunshine, helped me with my bags and saw me off at the dock. Au Revoir Ashram - off to Charlotte North Carolina, then Bettendorf, Arkansas to see John, Beatrice and Vivi. " (May 5 and 6)

So, after a year, What is Possible?

I've shared with you many of my physical and internal struggles, and noted changes that have occurred for me spiritually, mentally and physically along the way. The last section of this book provides before and after visuals as evidence of the physical changes. And while it would make for a perfect fairy tale ending to say that I found a wonderful life partner, as Elizabeth Gilbert did in her *Eat, Pray, Love* book, it is not the reality.

Surely, I was looking for love, as we all search for love, but I've found it in a very convenient place, inside me. I've grown that love to a greater capacity to encompass more people, as I work to be less judgmental and more patient, with myself and with others.

As I reflected and meditated in order to share the ultimate answer to my yearlong question of "What is Possible?", I believe the most important results are that I now think differently and feel differently than I did a year ago. I realize that to fix or change your life, your business, or the world, you have to start with yourself - and the single best way to change yourself is to focus on and help others. It seems counter-intuitive, and yet it works!

My inner self is much calmer and more peaceful. I have less fear and a better understanding of how to deal with the fears of the mind as they arise. I accept and acknowledge that fear, struggles and suffering will continue in life, and it's ok. I will adapt, adjust and accommodate as needed. I do not fear dying and I do not fear living. There is a greater freedom and ease to my outlook on life. I trust that there will be signals to guide me on the right path, and that tough obstacles may not mean that I am on the wrong path, just sidetracked perhaps for a lesson I need to learn. I have learned that I am not in control, except for choosing what karma will pave the path of my future. I am excited about creating good karma through kind, loving and generous thoughts and actions. With those actions, I will create a kind, loving and abundant future for myself and those around me.

Yogis teach that ultimately we are all on a spiritual quest, in search of experiencing the oneness of ourselves with God, as part of the universe and beyond. Yogis also teach that Love is at our core, and that our true nature is Bliss and Happiness.

My spirituality has been awakened, and I have observed the good, bad and ugly sides of my mind. I believe I have a long life ahead of me. As I face the inevitable challenges and struggles ahead, having a strong presence of God in my life and a disciplined yogic approach to my lifestyle will support me. I continue to train for the marathon of life. My daily living now includes the following practices: I wake and go to sleep with thoughts of God. I pause for gratitude and prayer at meal times. I daily practice yoga and chant Arati (a prayer), with a lit candle and incense whenever possible, to prepare the space I work in and write each day. I enjoy learning about and reading scriptures. I often mentally repeat my mantra, invoking God's name throughout my day, especially if I find myself feeling impatient or annoyed. The key is that these are all "practices", not goals or ways of being perfect. Each day I practice, and some days I do better than others, and it's all ok.

I now understand that it will require daily vigilance dedicated to my yoga practices to be a leader in life who is kind, loving and generous. It will be through living as my balanced and healthy self that I can be a leader who leads from the heart. My purpose in this lifetime is clear. It is simply to serve humanity. In my life, I've served as a daughter, a sister, a student, a friend, a mother, a wife, a teacher, a business and government employee, a business owner, a life coach, and now as a yoga teacher and writer. When I've brought my best self to my work, I have served humanity.

Gopi Kallayil carries two business cards. The one I particularly like reads *Happy Human*, Googler.

What is Possible? For me, it's being a healthier, more balanced **Happy Human!**

RESULTS

"Today, people are decaying, not aging.
The deficiency of awe and wonder is the greatest
deficiency today, and it leads to unhealthy aging."

Raphael Kellman, M.D.

Changes occurred throughout the year - some small and some pretty substantial. My Ayurvedic-Yogic approach to life, living a clean and healthy lifestyle, supported by spirituality and a focus on service to others, yielded some life-altering results.

Whether it was having the strength to open jars again, noticing improved hearing instead of further decline, having stable eyesight rather than the typical decline, the disappearance of cysts and no new cysts, having softened and healthy new skin, fewer aches in my joints or the many other improvements that were physical, emotional and spiritual - all of these changes can be attributed to adherence to the prescribed Ayurvedic -Yogic lifestyle.

An interesting email exchange took place on December 20th, as I reached out to KP with the following note:

"Om and Hi KP,

When we spoke, I meant to tell you of a really strange (to me) occurrence I've noticed the past couple of months - my breast tissue on the upper portion of my breast has refilled - the cleavage portion that had been sort of deflated without the enhancing effect of under garments has now reappeared as it was almost like new - hard to explain, but it is quite definitive and I have not gained weight - so it is not a weight gain phenomenon. And even when I was a bit heavier than I am now, my breast tissue was still older in appearance and the skin was not new, as it is now. As I write this, I realize I am not explaining it very well.

Anyway - it's great, except that all of my sports bras are now tight LOL"

KP's reply:

"That is very typical of the kinds of changes we see on a long-term program. Little things you did not expect to change get slowly better as you de-age."

I found the term quite fitting of my experiences over the year. It was like a 'de-aging' process, if we use the typical Western assumptions about aging.

One of the biggest changes for me, though, has been daily, healthy elimination without coffee. I've not had coffee for over a year, and I do not miss it. Besides the physically addictive nature of coffee, I came to realize there was also an emotional attachment, which centered around the social status and mainstream feel of the ritual. Drinking coffee somehow felt like a rite of passage into adulthood. Almost everyone I associated with drank coffee. I worried that my lifelong association with coffee, and with family and friends who drank coffee, would leave me feeling somehow out of touch with others and disassociation would follow.

Yet I've now become comfortable with the socialization that I thought would be the hardest part of giving it up. Nearly every coffee shop also has tea, and if they do not, hot water with lemon or plain hot water also works for me. I've come to realize that friendship and conversation is just as meaningful and fun with any drink of choice. Meeting for coffee and meeting for wine or alcoholic drinks was all habitual. It didn't occur to me that there were other ways to have relationships. I was attached to my familiar ways of thinking and learned way of doing things. I desired social engagements over coffee or over wine, margaritas, chocolate martinis, because I thought the drinks and venues were what made me happy and provided the fun!

I was wrong. The happiness comes from within.

Traditional Lab Test Results

The typical battery of tests in annual physicals have great value in medicine and in the treatment of many disorders, diseases and conditions. People benefit from the information in the tests, and doctors prescribe treatments based on the results. I'm not minimizing their value. Yet, something didn't add up for me.

- Where were the results that served as predictors of pending health issues?

- What test results were indicators of sleep deprivation?

- What test results provided insight about poor digestion?

- What test result indicated dryness of skin and loss of skin elasticity?

- Which results alerted the doctor and patient to increasing loss of strength, as in the inability to open a jar lid or lift a heavy item?

- What test would be an indicator of pending general discomfort and inability to find a relaxed and restful position to sit or sleep?

- What could these tests tell us about memory loss?

- What was the test for chronic constipation?

- Were there tests to prepare us for scalp cysts or muscle tension and joint inflammation?

As I mentioned earlier, when I suffered from the pinched nerves in the base of my spine, there were no other indicators present from blood or urine tests that showed me to be anything but healthy and in normal ranges for my age and gender. Tens of thousands of dollars were spent in search of relief from the pain and immobility. Yet not once was I asked about diet. I was asked about stress and work habits. When I said I had a stressful job at times, with many hours spent in front of the computer, it was acknowledged by the doctor as being a typical answer and accepted as a necessary requirement of the culture and the times. No suggestions for change in lifestyle were even considered by me or the doctors I saw - and I saw quite a few of them.

Also in the past, when I'd mentioned to doctors that I was often tired and didn't sleep well, the immediate response was this was normal as people age. Then the doctor inevitably offered to prescribe a drug for me to take. Throughout my life, I've refrained from taking prescription drugs, unless absolutely necessary for severe pain. I had no intention of taking drugs to fall asleep, and thus I always said 'no' to the prescription offers. My experience, though, and the experience of nearly everyone I know, is that drugs or surgery are the solutions to all issues when we go to a doctor in the U.S. It is part of the reason that Ayurveda intrigued me so much and also why I was open to alternative solutions for good health. Drugs and surgery just weren't registering with me as the optimal way to live life.

When I went in for a complete physical in 2015, before I left for the year in the Bahamas, my results showed me to be in normal ranges on all tests, with the exception of a Vitamin D deficiency.

This gave me baseline results for the study. I then had another complete physical when I returned home in May 2016, before leaving for Thailand.

The following are results comparisons from 2015 and 2016 physical exams and comments by KP Khalsa:

Diagnostic test	2015 (date)	2016 (date)	Comment
Glucose	83	77	Improvement - 83 was still very good
Protein	6.7	6.4	(low end of normal) This is not a measure of protein consumption or protein body level. It measures binding proteins in the blood. Range 6.4-8.3
Cholesterol	137	133	Minimal change 137 is already very low
HDL	63	61	Range 35 to 80 Change not significant (higher is better)
Cholesterol / HDL ratio	2.17 (good)	2.18 (good)	An optimal ratio is less than 3.5
LDL	63	62	Optimal less than 100
Triglycerides	57	51	Normal less than 150
Vitamin D	27 (low)	55 (good)	Range is 30-100, ideal 75

Commentary from *K P Khalsa*

The blood glucose measurement was initially quite good at 83, and ended the year at 77, which is essentially comparable. This is a sign of a generally good diet and overall level of health. The vast majority of Americans have high or unstable blood sugar. In America, metabolic syndrome (pre-diabetes) runs at about 35%. In those in their sixties and older, it is as high as 38% in women. Those people have a 22% higher mortality rate than people without pre-diabetes. For elders with both high blood sugar and high blood pressure, there is 82% higher mortality.

Cholesterol stayed in the same range, going from 137 to 133, an insignificant change. This is a very low number and would be considered by most cardiologists to be quite desirable. HDL, blood ratios, LDL and triglycerides all remained excellent, while the vitamin D level climbed from an unhealthy low of 27 to a very good level of 55.

A total serum protein test measures the total amount of protein in the blood. It also measures the amounts of two major groups of proteins in the blood: albumin and globulin. Albumin is made mainly in the liver. It helps keep the blood from leaking out of blood vessels. Albumin also helps carry some medicines and other substances through the blood and is important for tissue growth and healing. Globulin is made up of different proteins called alpha, beta, and gamma types. Some globulins are made by the liver, while others are made by the immune system. Certain globulins bind with hemoglobin. Other globulins transport metals, such as iron, in the blood and help fight infection. Serum globulin can be separated into several subgroups by serum protein electrophoresis.

Conventional medical tests are designed to find crises so that medical providers can respond to them. They are not designed to optimize a person's health, or even find every potential problem. Medical testing is a very blunt instrument. Also, most medical providers rarely, if ever, see a person in optimal health, or even a person who is aging in a healthy way. They are used to seeing people who are aging slowly, and poorly, so the norm is to chalk all that up to normal aging. Of course, those signs of degeneration are not normal, just typical, or average. As you have seen, the normal ranges in medical tests are quite broad, so that the far ends of the bell curve represent only truly sick people. Those people get attention and care, but sometimes the side effects of the treatments must be weighed against the benefits.

I daily noted about my sleeping and bowel movements in my journal, since two of the main imbalances I started out with were insomnia and irregular bowel movements. KP indicated to me that ideally, I would be sleeping 8 or more hours every night without the need to get up and go to the toilet, and my solid wastes would be eliminated upon rising in the morning. With the Ashram schedule, though, I regarded any night where I slept undisturbed for more than 5 hours as a full night's sleep, and most of my sound sleep nights were 6-7 hours of uninterrupted sleep.

In total, I logged 140 nights of more than 5 hours straight sleep, with 100 of the nights being between 6-7 hours of sound, undisturbed sleep. Considering where I started (only 2-3 hours of sleep at a time), this was a huge success for me. It's something I will continue to work on. It is not really surprising that the insomnia is taking some time to straighten out, as it has been an issue for me for over 40 years. The nights when I sleep 7 hours straight are incredible. I actually feel energetic and wide awake, and happy to get out of bed to start the day. This is not how I usually felt, or even feel now when I don't get a full night's rest. I've never considered myself a morning person, and in fact just the opposite. I always felt as if I was dragging myself out of bed each day, and the best thing about the morning for me was always coffee. I knew once I could get some coffee in me, I could wake up and face the day. Now, I have discovered that a little splash of water on my face or a shower works just as well as the coffee. I no longer drag myself out of bed, and the way I feel after a full night's rest has made it inconceivable for me to not work toward that same quality of sleep every night. It's truly worth it to feel more alive and energetic in the morning.

My waste elimination regularity, without coffee, was attained fairly quickly, from the perspective of having a bowel movement once a day. Within just a couple of months, I was having daily bowel movements. Having bowel movements upon rising in the morning, however, was not as easy. From Ayurveda's and KP's perspective, rising elimination was the ideal.

If I didn't sleep well, a 'first thing in the morning' solid waste evacuation was less frequent, and not of the quality and quantity of a healthy elimination. Without a good night's sleep, I tended to have small bowel movements (BMs) for my rising elimination, and then later in the morning had better evacuation. Generally, a good night's sleep also led to a rising BM. When I went through the count, I was surprised that the total number of rising BMs was the exact same number as the number of nights slept soundly. 140 mornings of rising with solid waste elimination - any size of elimination was considered success in this count. This was not a direct correlation, but the results are still very interesting.

I'll continue to work on having rising BMs, but I can share that just having daily solid waste evacuation is a blessing and makes such a difference in how I feel throughout the day. I can't believe how many years I went without this very basic functioning of the body working properly.

My list of issues when this study began:

- **Vitamin D deficiency - identified in the baseline physical exam**
  Resolved

- **Erratic sleeping - and had periods of hot and cold each night**
  Temperature Fluctuations Resolved, Longer Periods of Sleeping with increased regularity

- **Constipation and difficult bowel movements**
  Resolved

- **Cracked, sore and dry skin, especially on feet**
  No soreness, dryness and cracks minimal and continue to improve

- **Loss of elasticity in skin, especially face but also body**
  Skin texture and overall appearance of the skin is improved and new skin is being generated beyond what I expected

- **Scalp cysts**
  Resolved

- **Thinning hair and eyelashes**
  Both hair and eyelashes have new growth and continue to be fuller and thicker

- **Receding hairline**
  New growth of hair rather than further recession

- **Right knee pain and sensitivity**
  Still some discomfort at times, but is no longer a real issue

- **Left big toe nail was not growing and had been damaged for more than 10 years**
  Nail is growing - it's very slow but continues to improve

- **Toes starting to grow crooked and bunions forming**
  Toes are straightening and bunions are slowly receding

- **Neck pain and stiffness from prior whiplash car accident**
  This issue is still in progress. There has been improvement, but it is not resolved.

- **Stiffness in shoulder area**
  Very little problem with my shoulder now - mostly feels good and better range of motion

- **Finger nails discolored, yellowing and white spots and ridges**
  Resolved and healthy, pink tone to skin under nails, no spots and ridges are nearly completely gone

- **Bloating**
  Much better

- **Gasses passed often and with foul odor**
  Rarely foul odor and less frequent passing of gas

- **Belching after meals**
  Resolved as long as I eat appropriately - not too fast and not overeating

- **Left ear hearing loss steadily declining**
  Incredible improvement in hearing that I never expected - not full hearing like my right ear, but great improvement

- **Strength in hands declining - could not open jars for a few years**
  Improved strength and can open jars, continual improvement over the year

- **Memory was declining**
  I feel that my mind faculties have been sharpened

- **Difficulty finding comfortable sitting position and also sleeping position - very fidgety and rarely at peace**
  Continually improving

- **Frequent urination throughout the day and at night**
  Much improved from where I was

In Thailand, focused on writing and away from the controlled, supportive environment of the Ashram, I continued to notice physical improvements. The skin on the bottoms of my feet continued to improve and show new growth, while my big toenail continued to slowly improve. My hair also continued to thicken, with eyelashes, body and scalp hair all showing signs of growth.

RESULTS - COMMENTARY

By *K P Khalsa*

Padmavati is primarily pitta constitution, which is why she was drawn to the hard-charging professional world, and was good at it. Because of her stage of life, and the consequences of her lifestyle, her imbalances at the start of her year were virtually all from aggravated vata. Insomnia, declining strength, waning memory, constipation, inflexible skin, joint stiffness, sensory loss and hair changes are all vata symptoms. Better hearing and more mobile joints do not seem like they mean you're not about to have a heart attack, but, in fact, they are a general indication of improving health that makes a crisis much less likely.

Padmavati's improvement in all these areas, while probably appreciated by a medical doctor, would have no effect on the doctor's thinking. Likely they would be deemed coincidence. But we know from yoga that these developments all signal that vata is retreating, and we know from millennia of experience that this means a much more comfortable elder hood. Why be sick and declining for twenty years, and then die slowly, begging for the release from the body, like most people today?

During this year, which is just the beginning, from an Ayurveda point of view, we concentrated on aggressively controlling the heightened vata. Over time, while still managing these vata issues, she will need to gradually transition to slow acting anti-aging, tonic remedies that extend life, improve physical comfort, promote mental stability and enhance immune function.

Many of the issues that plagued Padmavati were not life threatening or in the nature of a crisis. Poor sleep, who doesn't have that? Bowel movements, who cares? But imagine simply waking each day feeling great. Wouldn't that be a wonderful gift? Having nice skin is not a requirement for a happy life, though you certainly would prefer it.

Even if you think of these issues as minor irritations, they signify an advancing tidal wave of vata dosha, the destructive principle. Maybe if vata killed us quickly, we could discount it. But the slow, miserable decline these signs portend is the kicker. Most of us do not want an elder hood like our parents, slowly grinding to a halt, breaking a hip and grimly expiring while every effort is made to extend our life, but not our vibrancy.

Taking on an Ayurvedic perspective at any time of life will help you wind back the clock and also help you avoid developing the truly devastating diseases that make people in our culture miserable—diabetes, heart disease and cognitive decline.

I can't tell you how many people have told me they did not realize they had bad digestion until they got good digestion. Or substitute any body part, system or symptom. We see everyone around us suffering, so it seems normal. This silent suffering was not always the case. In earlier generations, people's problems ended to be acute, such as a drastic infection or a traumatic accident. On a day-to-day basis, people got refreshing sleep, digested their food and had regular bowel habits. The change to today's enigma was so gradual that almost no one noticed. Your friends are constipated, tired and on the brink of a cold most of the time, so it must be normal, right? Not so! As you have read, Padmavati proved that having vigor, energy and comfort is our natural condition. We just have to make some decisions and stick to them. I have never seen anyone who has done so regret it.

The photos that follow are "before and after" shots, taken just before I started the year at the Ashram, and again just before I left. I took similar photos each month, with the kind assistance of numerous karma yogis. The differences from month to month were less obvious, but the full year comparisons are quite significant in the amount of change that can be seen.

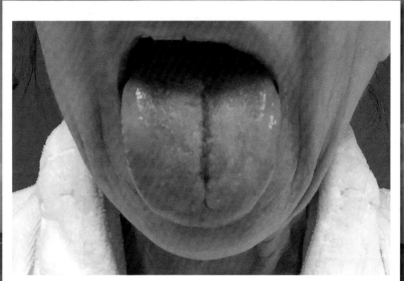

Tongue Before

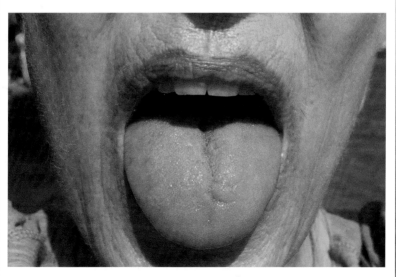

Tongue After

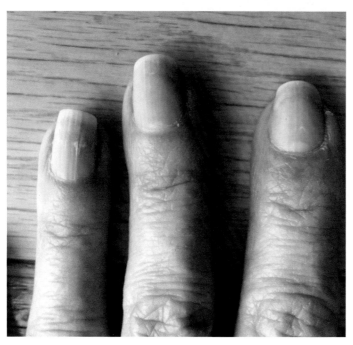

Fingernails Before

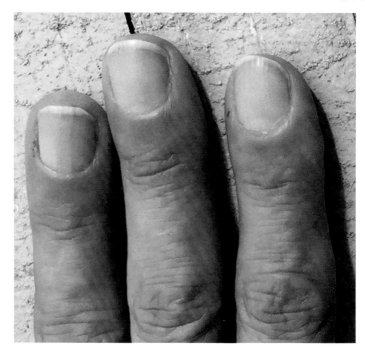

Fingernails After

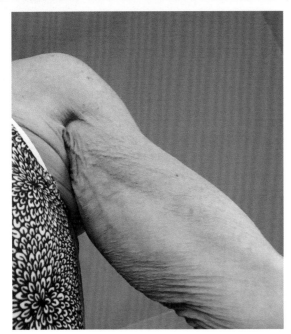

Arms Before

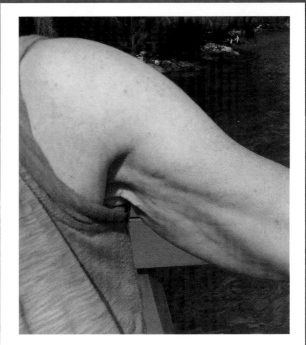

Arms After

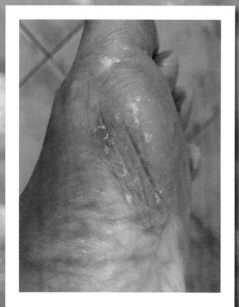

Foot Before

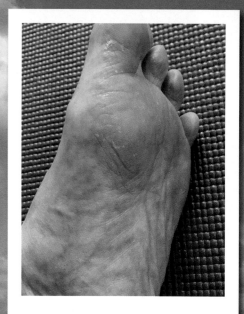

Foot After

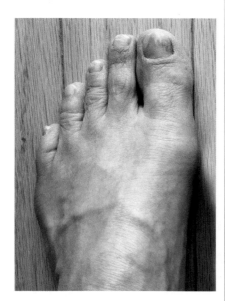

*Before
Toes Crooked &
Bunion Forming*

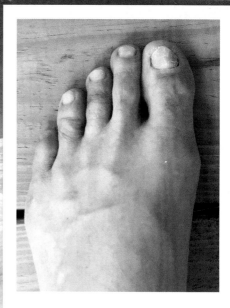

*After
Straighter Toes &
Bunion Receding*

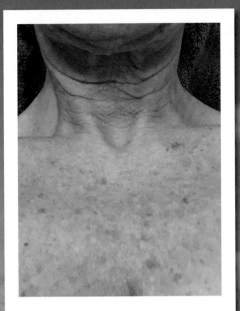

Neck/Chest Before

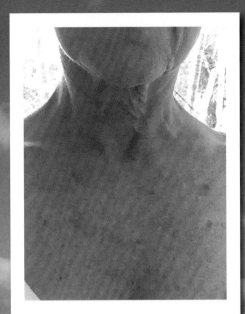

Neck/Chest After

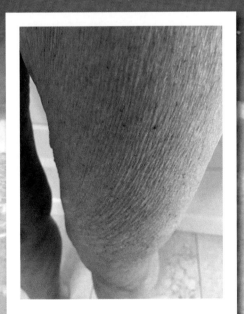

Thigh Before

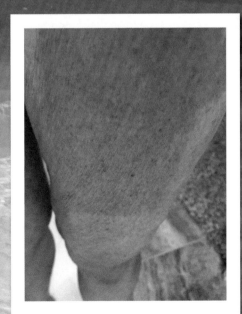

Thigh After

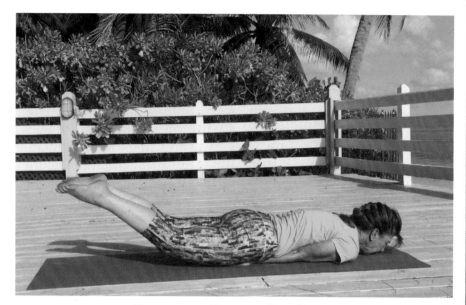

Locust Pose Before

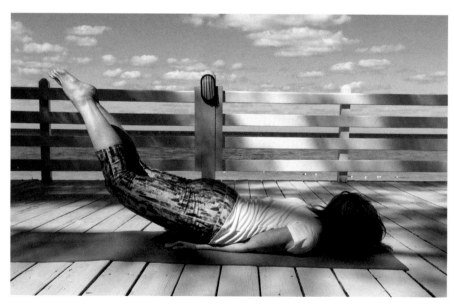

Locust Pose After

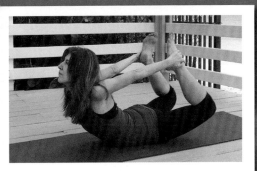

Bow Pose Before

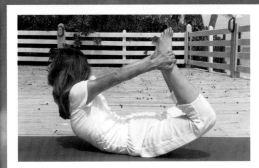

Bow Pose After

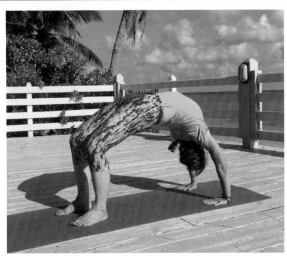

Backbend Before

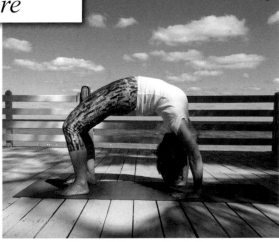

Backbend After

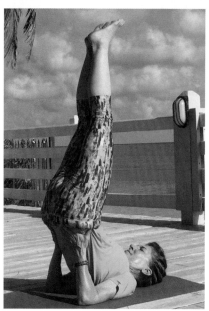

Shoulder Stand
Before

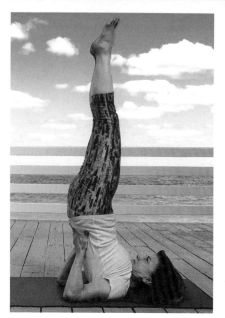

Shoulder Stand
After

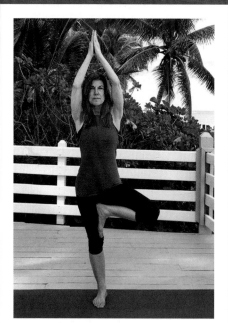

Tree Pose
Before

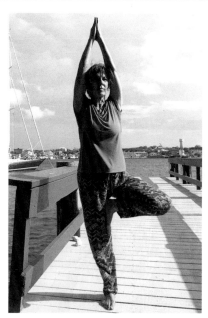

Tree Pose
After

RESOURCES

Ayurveda

KP Khalsa, Ayurveda Doctor (AD) - KP leads the International Integrative Educational Institute as one of the foremost natural healing experts in North America. KP is an internationally known speaker and has written and shared a wealth of articles on his website and written a number of excellent books, including his latest and my favorite, *The Way of Ayurvedic Herbs*. He also teaches accreditation programs in Herbalist Training and Ayurveda and offers a wide selection of webinars to help us all learn more about health issues and solutions that are natural and effective, yet easy to follow. He shares in simple language, what herbs to take and what they are good for. **www.kpkhalsa.com**

Banyan Botanicals - Certified organic, sustainably sourced and fairly traded herbs **www.banyanbotanicals.com**

Dr. Deepak Chopra - Co-creator of the Chopra Center in Carlsbad, California, wrote the book *Perfect Health*, which was my entry level book to Ayurveda. I believe it to be a good foundational book for someone newly interested in alternative approaches to healing. The Chopra Center website also has many articles and lots of great information. **www.chopra.com**

Dr. Vasant Lad - Director of the Ayurvedic Institute in Albuquerque, New Mexico, teaches accreditation programs, lectures worldwide and has a vast amount of information on his website. One of my favorite of his books, *Ayurveda, The Science of Self Healing,* is quite helpful for someone interested in learning more about Ayurveda. **www.ayurveda.com**

Yoga

Sivananda Ashram Yoga Retreat (SAYR) - The Sivananda Ashram in the Bahamas has a very informative website and some great programs. Whether you are interested in a yoga retreat vacation or taking an accreditation healing therapy course or taking the yoga teacher training course, SAYR is a great place to explore and consider. You can also subscribe to their blog, which often carries some of our favorite recipes. **www.sivanandabahamas.org**

Swami Sivananda and Swami Vishnudevananda - Master Swami Sivananda and his disciple, Swami Vishnudevananda offered the world teachings through a variety of books. Swami Sivananda wrote nearly 400 books, and one of my favorites is *Bliss Divine*. Swami Sivananda's books are free to download from The Divine Life Society, which he founded. **www.dlshq.org/download/download.htm**

Swami Vishnudevananda wrote the *Complete Illustrated Book of Yoga*, which is the foundation book for the yoga Teacher Training Course at the Ashram. This book is an invaluable resource for a yoga teacher. The book can be purchased through Amazon or at the Sivananda Ashrams and Centers worldwide.

The Divine Life Society - This organization was founded by Swami Sivananda. It has many articles and a wealth of information about meditation, pranayama and all things yoga. **www.sivanandaonline.org**

Mentioned in the Book:

Joan Borysenko - Best selling author and speaker has a wealth of information on her site **www.joanborysenko.com**

California College of Ayurveda - Dr. Marc Halpern is the founder of this Ayurveda training college. There is a wealth of information on the website **www.ayurvedacollege.com**

Kam Thye Chow - Thai Yoga Massage **www.kamthyechow.com**

Karnamarita Dasi - Beautiful songstress and chanter, Karnamarita's website also has schedules of her upcoming events besides her music **www.dasimusic.com**

Dr. Joe Dispenza - A number of Books, including Amazon and New York Best Seller, *You Are the Placebo: Making Your Mind Matter*, DVDs, lectures, classes, events - all can be found on international speaker and neuroscientist, Dr. Joe's website **www.drjoedispenza.com**

John Douillard - Books, DVD's, courses all can be found on the LifeSpa website, the company he founded **www.lifespa.com**

Dr. Daniel Drubach - Dr. Drubach has an extensive list of publications, interests and general bio information on his Mayo Clinic web page. **www.mayoclinic.org/ biographies/drubach-daniel-a-m-d/bio-20053352**

iRest Yoga Nidra - Richard Miller and Molly Birkholm - Worldwide trainings and a wealth of information can be found on the website **www.irest.us** Richard is the founder of iRest and can be found on the iRest website. Molly Birkholm has yoga nidra CDs and other information about Warriors at Ease, a post traumatic stress disorder program for veterans she co-founded, on her Healing River website **www.healingriveryoga.com**

Gopi Kallayil - Gopi's latest book, *The Internet to the Inner-Net* is full of personal stories from his work at Google to his travels around the world. He has some practical tips for bringing your life and your company to a more conscious state. **www.kallayil.com**

Sat Bir Singh Khalsa - Harvard researcher and teacher **www.yoga-research.info/ satbirsinghkhalsa.html**

Landmark - The organization that leads transformational education programs that bring about breakthroughs in personal and professional lives **www.landmark-worldwide.com**

Tao Porchon Lynch - Tao also has a recent book about her life, an autobiography, *Dancing Light*. Yoga class schedules, lectures and inspiration can be found on her website. She continues to teach yoga and compete in dance competitions. **www. taoporchon-lynch.com**

Father William Meninger - Father Meninger can be found on a couple of websites, and his recent book, *The Process of Forgiveness*, is sold on Amazon, **www.contemplativeprayer.net** and **www.contemplativeprayerdotnet.wordpress.com**

Aadil Palkhivala - Author of *Fire of Love,* an inspiring book with stories of yoga and devoted to Sri Aurobindo's methodology **www.aadil.com**

John Perkins - New York Times Best Selling author of *Confessions of an Economic Hitman*, activist, Chief Economist **www.johnperkins.org**

G.S. Sachdev - Beautiful classical music master, playing the Bansuri flute with master Swapan Chaudhuri accompanying on the tabla **www.gssachdev.wordpress.com**

Shimshai - Music and tour schedule can be found on his website **www.shimshai.com**

Dr. Michael Spezio - Dr. Spezio has a long list of research and publications on his web page. **www.scrippscollege.edu/academics/faculty/profile/michael-spezio**

Sri Aurobindo - Yogi, guru, philosopher **www.sriaurobindoashram.org/ashram/ sriauro/life_sketch.php**

Tejas Yoga Studio (Chicago) - **www.tejasyogachicago.com**

Gaura Vani & As Kindred Spirits - Kirtan music and chants can be downloaded from this site **www.gauravani.com**

GRATITUDE

Each of the following people encouraged, guided, supported, taught, inspired and enriched my life in ways that helped to surface my truth as I embarked on this yearlong study.

For life itself and a loving environment to grow up in, I am grateful to my parents. They were my first teachers. They gave of themselves, so that I and my brothers could have opportunities they did not have. I was blessed to always be surrounded by a supportive family. Thank You!

My children, their spouses and my grandchildren are also blessings, for which I am thankful. They've encouraged me and supported me throughout this journey. And, through the wonders of technology, they've shared their lives with me via videos, FaceTime and photos, even when we've been thousands of miles apart. My heart was filled with each sharing. Thank You!

My partner, KP Khalsa, took a chance on me and this study, from a place of faith and his true interest in healing the world. He taught me through his open and selfless acceptance of my proposal, that saying 'yes' to a crazy proposal from a total stranger can lead to a wonderful partnership. I am grateful for his strong faith, his deep expertise, his time, his dedication to healing, his humor and his patience. It has been an honor and a privilege to work together with him as a team. Thank You!

My host and partner, Sivananda Ashram Yoga Retreat, under the leadership of Swami Swaroopananda and Swami Prema, welcomed me with open arms and provided an amazing, spiritually charged environment for my yearlong journey. I was fortunate to have had such beauty surrounding me and a spiritually rich place to live. Each of the senior staff, and especially Rukmini, my supervisor, supported me and taught me life altering lessons. I am very grateful for Rukmini's love and guidance, and for the embrace of the entire senior staff, who also guided and watched over me. Swami Brahmananda, Nirmala and Satyadev, Krishnadas and Swami Hridyananda were my Teacher Training Course instructors - the TTC experience and teachings are gifts I will treasure for the rest of my life. Thank you!

Banyan Botanicals was a great partner and immense help, so that I was able to use high quality herbs and supplements for the study. I am very grateful for their willingness to support my study and their sincere interest in helping people to have alternative choices for their medicinal needs, by providing all natural, high quality products. Thank You!

Lotus Press entered my world, unsuspectingly and felt like a gift straight from God. I am blessed and grateful for their willingness to publish and print *What's Possible?* It is my sincere hope that our efforts as a team will influence the world, for the better. Thank You!

Rukmini Ali Shevlin, my editor, has been an amazing partner during the writing process. Her forthright and yet encouraging approach were exactly what I needed to continue to improve and revise the writing, while keeping the flow of creativity alive. Her keen intuitive sense helped to guide me in the direction I wanted to go, while helping me to get there with finesse and grace. She truly is a gifted editor and was a joy to work with. I was blessed by her support and treasure her friendship. I know the book is better because of our working on it together. Thank You!

My 'Readers' gave of their time, by reading the full DRAFT of the book and are greatly appreciated. Sri Devi Jennie Hastings, Sandy Jones, Amanda Landsman, Justin Landsman, Maheshwari Karen Maloney, Mary Ellen Middleton, David Vaught and KP Khalsa helped to make the book better for a wide range of audience. Their feedback was invaluable and sparked much revision. Thank You!

My proofreader, Sri Devi Jennie Hastings, gave her time and dedication to detail, as she read to find the mistakes that escaped me and my editor. Her work greatly helped to refine the writing and ready it for it's final draft to be sent to the publisher. Thank You!

James Tenant, Jim Bennitt and the Tejas Yoga Community helped prepare and open me up for the healing that took place during the yearlong study. I am grateful for their love, support and dedication to yoga. Introducing me to the spiritual side of yoga, pranayama and Ayurveda were the sparks that ignited my interest and longing to learn more. Thank You!

Jillmarie and Takemitsu Kawaoka, your love and your Christmas gift, *How Yoga Works* by Geshe Michael Roach, challenged my thinking about life itself. Then you shared Landmark Forum and the other Landmark courses with me, and I was again intrigued and challenged. I appreciate having had each of these opportunities to reframe my thinking and shake some of the cobwebs of my life up a bit. My deep love and respect for you gave me the faith I needed to try out these new ideas. I'm so glad that I did. Thank You!

Longtime friends and BestYOU followers have supported me from afar, reading my blog posts and sending me notes of encouragement throughout the year. I am deeply grateful to you for the positive energy you sent my way. Thank You!

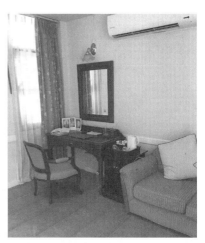

New friends that I've made in Thailand, from Chiang Dow to Chiang Mai, have made my solo trip here much more fun. The wonderful friends I met in Thailand from the US and UK, the staff at Eurasia hotel, the owner of Aum restaurant, the familiar, always smiling faces of the Thai people in the shops, markets and cafes - all were my family away from home. They played an integral part in my overall emotional and mental state, as relation-ships are the best way to express and receive love. I felt love the entire three months that I was in Thailand. Thank You!

And to each of YOU, thank you very much for taking this journey with me and for being here right now. Namaste.

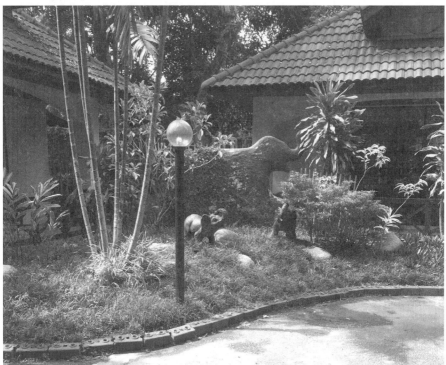

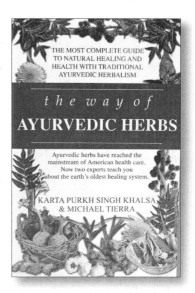